Health Research in Practice

Research in Practice

Health Research in Practice

Political, ethical and methodological issues

Edited by

Derek Colquhoun

*School of Education, Deakin University,
Geelong, Australia*

Allan Kellehear

*Department of Sociology, La Trobe University,
Bundoora, Australia*

CHAPMAN & HALL

London · Glasgow · New York · Tokyo · Melbourne · Madras

Published by Chapman & Hall, 2–6 Boundary Row, London SE1 8HN

Chapman & Hall, 2–6 Boundary Row, London SE1 8HN, UK

Blackie Academic & Professional, Wester Cleddens Road, Bishopbriggs, Glasgow G64 2NZ, UK

Chapman & Hall Inc., 29 West 35th Street, New York NY10001, USA

Chapman & Hall Japan, Thomson Publishing Japan, Hirakawacho Nemoto Building, 6F, 1–7–11 Hirakawa-cho, Chiyoda-ku, Tokyo 102, Japan

Chapman & Hall Australia, Thomas Nelson Australia, 102 Dodds Street, South Melbourne, Victoria 3205, Australia

Chapman & Hall India, R. Seshadri, 32 Second Main Road, CIT East, Madras 600 035, India

Distributed in the USA and Canada by Singular Publishing Group Inc., 4284 41st Street, San Diego, California 92105

First edition 1993

© 1993 Chapman & Hall

Typeset in 10/12 Palatino by Mews Photosetting, Beckenham, Kent
Printed in England by Clays Ltd., St. Ives plc

ISBN 0 412 47470 0   1 56593 143 2 (USA)

A catalogue record for this book is available from the British Library

Library of Congress Cataloging-in-Publication data
Health research in practice : political, ethical, and methodological
    issues / edited by Derek Colquhoun, Allan Kellehear. – 1st ed.
        p. cm.
    Includes index.
    ISBN 0-412-47470-0 (acid-free paper)
        I. Public health–Research–Methodology. I. Colquhoun. Derek.
    II. Kellehear, Allan.
    RA440.85.H43 1993
    362.1′072–dc20   93-7072
                                                          CIP

∞ Printed on permanent acid-free text paper, manufactured in accordance with the proposed ANSI/NISO Z 39.48-199X and ANSI Z 39.48-1984

For Jessie and Bill Colquhoun

Contents

Contributors

Derek Colquhoun Lecturer in Education, Deakin University, Geelong, Australia

Jeanne Daly Research Fellow in Sociology, La Trobe University, Bundoora, Australia

Ann Daniel Associate Professor of Sociology, University of New South Wales, Kensington, Australia

Liz Eckermann Lecturer in Sociology, Deakin University, Geelong, Australia

Michael Gliksman Research Fellow in Epidemiology, University of Sydney, Sydney, Australia

Allan Kellehear Senior Lecturer in Sociology, La Trobe University, Bundoora, Australia

Robin McTaggart Associate Professor of Education, Deakin University, Geelong, Australia

Chris Peterson Lecturer in Applied Sociology, Swinburne University of Technology, Hawthorn, Australia

Ian Robottom Senior Lecturer in Education, Deakin University, Geelong, Australia

Lynne Stevens Postgraduate in Education, Deakin University, Geelong, Australia

Bev Taylor Senior Lecturer in Nursing, Deakin University, Geelong, Australia

Rob Walker Professor of Education, Deakin University, Geelong, Australia

Evan Willis Senior Lecturer in Sociology, La Trobe University, Bundoora, Australia

Preface

The past few years have witnessed an important rethink about the way we approach health research. For example, three major journals in the health area, *Health Education: Theory and Practice*, *Health Education Quarterly* and *Social Science and Medicine*, have recently devoted special issues to qualitative methodologies. Increasingly researchers are questioning the conventional wisdom and assumptions that have been the traditional foundations of research practice in health. This practice has been dominated by concerns about 'technique' and a seemingly endless obsession with validity, reliability and generalizability. These questions are not unimportant but neither are they all important. Their dominance in books about health research however, does have an unfortunate consequence for the area as a whole. It deflects attention away from other important issues within the research process. The aim of this book is to address these 'other' issues, issues which not only balance prevailing perspectives but, indeed, contextualize them.

For us, the term 'methods' merely implies techniques. These are concerns about abstract possibilities in ideal conditions. They are discussions which occur away from the human relationships and social processes of the research act itself. On the other hand, methodological discussions, which are our concern in this book, cover ontological and epistemological issues. These 'other' issues in health research ask questions about what it means to be a researcher and also the nature of knowledge itself. This is not a navel gazing exercise. The fact is, the less each of us understands our research preconceptions the more will we be blindly driven and constrained by them. Focusing on the research process allow us to see how politics and ethics are actually reflections of each other. It also allows us to see more clearly how other people – co-researchers, employers, peer cultures and 'the researched' – determine the research experience far more critically and deeply than do abstract principles of 'design' learnt in classroom situations. Health research, as presented in this book, is not simply practice, but also lived-in-experience, an experience which is formative as well as acted upon. This idea of the formative nature of research experience is the underlying theme of the book and, we believe, distinguishes it from other treatise which view research as 'something we do to others'.

This latter image of researcher as actor and the researched as audience is misleading, particularly for new researchers. When they consult conventional texts on methods they discover all too quickly that those texts have been sanitized. Researchers have edited themselves out of their accounts, reports and textbooks. Even more than this, the complex politics of the research process, the formative and active influences on 'the researcher' by the many others that he or she encounters have also been edited out of these texts.

In the following chapters, the contributors discuss the complexities of their own examples of health research. The personal and professional perspectives blend rather than hide from one another. These are not simply personal 'tales form the field'. Rather they are discussions about the relationship between research and researched, the politics of practice, the applications of certain methods in theory and practice. These discussions engage and interrogate other literature on the subject, but they also base their discussion on personal accounts of the research experience. Ideas and experience, theory and practice, question each other.

Daniel begins the collection by describing her experience in researching a dispute between doctors, bureaucrats and politicians. She walked a delicate political and ethical tightrope which highlights many of the dilemmas of research in health. She reflects on the research process and proposes some principles of good practice which emerged from that experience. Gliksman details similar problems. Squeezed between management and trade union hostilities, Gliksman describes the steps he took to produce research which would be honest to all parties, including himself. These steps include the need for a literature review, an independent management structure, a consideration of the advantages and disadvantages of available study designs, and the need for confidentiality.

Daly and Peterson continue with their more formal concerns with the interpersonal politics of health research. Daly discusses interdisciplinary health research involving clinicians and sociologists and in particular she illustrates the negotiation process for changing the rules of clinical research so that sociologists can contribute their special skills to the research. Peterson reflects on teaching health research in a non-social science context. He demonstrates how using methodologically familiar practices for physical sciences can also serve as preliminary steps to introducing more qualitative work. Colquhoun and Robottom reflect on more subtle and less obvious issues of politics and power in research by discussing issues of empowerment in participatory action research. This is extended by McTaggart's provocative and incisive chapter on similar issues in participatory action research in cross-cultural contexts. McTaggart draws on two examples, one from health education in the Sudan and one from Aboriginal teacher education in Australia to discuss some of the substantive, ethical and political issues in cross-cultural participatory action research.

Willis, Taylor and Kellehear discuss the historical, phenomenological and survey method respectively. Willis argues for a greater role in health research for the historical sociological method. He outlines some of the practical lessons that emerged from his research. Taylor looks at the phenomenological method in the theory and practice of nursing research. She reflects on her PhD research experience and suggests that the tension between idealized representations of the research process and the reality of researching a given context often necessitates a flexibility of approach and expectations. Kellehear asks us to have another look at the survey method of interviewing. Using an example from his research with terminally ill cancer sufferers Kellehear shows how he responded, not to favourite methodological dispositions, but rather to the unique circumstances and health of his respondents.

Walker looks at the problems of evaluation research in health, a method whose star is rising in the healthcare world. Walker sets us the considerable challenge of rethinking this thing called evaluation, particularly some of the deeply inscribed assumptions about policy, practice and bureaucratic structures. Stevens and Eckermann both discuss what it means to do health research within a feminist framework, and they come to different but complementary conclusions. They argue that there is no end to problems. One learns from ongoing reflexivity, imagination and experience. Stevens' chapter highlights this reflexivity, imagination and experience through the recounting of her Honours research in health education through a 'confessional tale'. Eckerman reflects on her research with women and eating disorders to illustrate some of the many substantive concerns in the eating disorder area and also to question many of the traditional methodological issues in health research. That style of reflection and sharing of our research experiences is the hallmark of this book. These narratives restore a political and social context to health research which, by their very union, allow us to see more clearly where the important challenges in this area lie.

Derek Colquhoun and Allan Kellehear

CHAPTER 1

Politicians, bureaucrats and the doctors: researching in the crossfire

Ann Daniel

LEARNING AND RESEARCH

Engaging in a major research project is likely to teach more about the art of research than can be gained from years of diligent attention to book learning. The continuing recurrence of this experience underlines the standing of the PhD as the traditional rite of passage for entry into academe. Such a proposition about the pedagogical value of field research does not in any way devalue the scholarship essential to any intellectually driven enterprise, but stresses that empirical inquiry enlivens theory and links it to practical issues. For me such a major research project developed from a traditional line of scholarly enquiry which had captured my intermittent attention for some years. I had been engaged in a critical examination of the literature on professions, searching for answers to questions prompted by observation of professionals at work and by my own participatory observation of academic teaching and research. This led through some serendipitous events to the research which is described in *Medicine and the State* (Daniel, 1990). In this chapter I will reflect on instructive aspects of that research process and abstract some principles of good practice which emerged from that experience.

My interest in professions had been aroused by earlier research concerned with prestige of occupations (Daniel, 1983). This had confirmed the continued high status of professions and pointed to the cultural and material bases of that standing. But that study revealed nothing about the way professions had come to secure and exploit those bases nor of the strategies which maintained professional sovereignty or dominance. Furthermore the review of professions formed only a small part of that study and anything more had to be put aside until later. That work in the late 1970s was for my doctorate and I, like most PhD students, was confronted with a host of observations, ideas and interpretations that must be excluded from the thesis and followed at a later date. After a number of other projects (some productive, some not) I returned to study the traditional professions.

The project, which I then planned, concentrated on three professions and was bent on discovering the distinctive features, resources and strategies adopted by each. Comparative studies can help the researcher to escape from the specificities of one case study; the inevitable contrasts can produce answers of greater validity and generalizability. I had spent some time learning the language and familiarizing myself with the general perspectives, the dominant paradigms, of accountancy, medicine and law. I had determined the questions that would guide the project, all concerned with the strategies that secure and hold a monopoly control of a lucrative and prestigious field. But there were practical problems. How could I enter the field and observe professional practice? What access might I be allowed to reports, records and other documents held by professional associations? Would I be allowed to attend committee meetings concerned with the issues – political, financial, ethical – which confront occupational associations and unions most of the time? Who would give time to answering my questions? This last was the most obdurate problem; most practitioners were in private practice and reluctant to give time to the data-collecting sociologist. I was exploring ways into the field when the unexpected happened.

OPPORTUNITY AND FLEXIBILITY

It was late in 1983 and discontent was growing in the hospitals. The grumbling distrust endemic in relations between doctors and government sharpened as their disagreements multiplied and intensified. The Federal Government was urging rationalization of health services, especially the expensive hospital services which it subsidized through the state governments. While the Federal Government provides the bulk of the funds in Australia, it is the State Governments in their local areas that provide most of the services (police, roads, schools, hospitals and so on). As part of the planning for control and rationalization the conditions governing private practice in public hospitals were to be altered. This struck at the nature of medical practice in Australia and threatened professional autonomy, authority and income. The medical profession was gravely alarmed and its leaders took up entrenched positions. As the dispute escalated I changed the focus of my research and concentrated on the medical profession and its arguments with Federal and State Governments.

In the turmoil engendered by debates and confrontations people were now willing, even eager, to put forward their points of view. They found time to speak and ensure that proceedings were open to a sociologist who 'should know what the real issues are and keep the record straight'. No request for an interview was refused.

In the ensuing excitement a principle which can be easily overlooked emerged. It is the first of those I will highlight in these reflections on the research process:

1. *In times of rapid change or conflict the inherent character of institutions becomes salient and their material and ideal interests are pursued more vigorously – Emile Durkheim had explained that in such times the bonds that indicate the interdependencies typical of society are stretched tight and become 'visible'. This is a very good time for research.*

DIRECT FUNDING

The changing pace of events had demanded a rapid response and what had been a fairly leisurely research exercise changed direction and gathered momentum. My teaching load for those early months of 1984 was heavy and I would not be able to interview the many participants, the factional leaders of all 'sides' drawn into the fracas. I appealed to the Dean and was immediately allocated a small grant to employ a part-time assistant. Val Russell and I set out to record the spoken values, opinions, expectations and determinations of all involved. Val had recently completed a BA (Hons) thesis on changes in public administration in the New South Wales state health services and was a highly perceptive interviewer. She was informed and sensitive to the issues and people readily entrusted to her their version of the individual and collective interests at stake. There are more lessons in this; the first goes to flexibility in funding:

2. *Research opportunities in the social sciences can appear suddenly and are best supported by small, immediate funding. The universities are qualified and well placed to assess and fund such opportunities.*

INFORMED TEAM WORK

Interviewers intent on eliciting relatively comprehensive and informative responses should be acquainted with the issues that concern those respondents and should know the structure of the institutions that they plan to explore. This is, of course, not an expectation that the interviewer knows the answers. In this case the research was well served by interviewers already informed about the structure of the recently established New South Wales Health Department, its functions and responsibilities; about the organization of the Australian Medical Association; the specialist associations and other groups representing sectional medical interests; about the hospital as the healthcare institution and the way its medical services were organized. The necessity for being well briefed before commencing an investigation is not one which I would extend to research of a more positivist nature where the interviewer acts largely as a channel of communication between the researcher and the researched, where a set of preconceived, precoded questions are put to the respondent. That approach has its proper place in large-sample surveys devised to obtain information and tap a set range of easily articulated opinions. The study whose lessons are here being recapitulated was of a different character. Where the researcher is seeking an understanding of what drives the activities and strategies that people adopt, what constitutes the interests, ideals and values being served and why events turn out the way they do, all of the research team should become familiar with the issues and the organizations under study before engaging in interviews with the participants. In health research there is available a wealth of documents setting out organisational missions, policies and regulations; there are press statements and media reports of intentions, decisions and initiatives; controversial issues prompt public meetings, demonstrations, debates in parliament. For the imaginative researcher the list of reports and events which can be accessed extends as the study continues. In health research there is rarely any excuse for uninformed interviewing; this points to a third aspect to be considered at the beginning:

3. *Research aimed at comprehensive and finely detailed interpretation of what is happening and what it all means to those involved requires a careful study of the issues, the social structures and their cultural and political context, before any of the researchers enters the field and starts asking questions.*

EFFECTIVE TEAM WORK

The fourth point is closely related to the third which assumes being informed and sharing that information within the team. It comes from the experience known to many sociologists of working in good and bad teams. The goodness or badness is not derived from the character or ability of the investigators, but from both their theoretical orientation and the priority they give the project. Sociological and political research of health-related issues cannot be atheoretical if it is to engender understanding, or explanation, of policies, practices and outcomes in the health field. Some theoretical diversity can be productive, but if researchers operate out of different paradigms co-operative effort will be frustrated. Researchers engaged on the one project should work out and agree on basic premises and objectives. This is not an argument against interdisciplinary teams which can co-operate productively, but a note about reconciling theoretical differences in the beginning. The myth of the Tower of Babel is instructive.

More patently relevant is the priority given to a project by each researcher; this should be made explicit. The urgency with which each approaches the research tasks can and will vary and the relative contribution and productivity of each member may differ. These matters should be recognized and agreed, at least tacitly, from the beginning and can be reviewed and resolved as necessary. Freeloaders have no place in a team; the effect on morale alone can be devastating. The caution should be acknowledged in the proposition:

4. A small research team engaged in the field together and consulting frequently increases the effectiveness of their work exponentially; the synergy can be remarkable. If the collective energies are being dissipated by disregard, disagreements and divergencies, review quickly and consider ways of dividing the project into discrete parts for sole players; if dissipation persists prepare to abandon the project.

THEORY AND THE DIALECTICS OF THEORIZING

In my view this is the most important and often the most difficult aspect of health research. Too much research in health and medicine is empiricist – narrow and superficial. Good research generates broader understanding of human action and the social structures it encounters and produces, of the resistance of the social and cultural to both individual and group action. From the complex and chaotic interplay of human intentionality and action, research can abstract interpretations, even explanations, that can be generalized beyond the immediate contingencies of one set of conditions.

The investigation of the doctors' dispute had stemmed from a more general inquiry into professions and their strategies for winning and holding control of valued and lucrative fields of practice. With the rapid escalation of conflict between the medical profession and the state the direction of the research had changed radically. Still about professions and processes of domination, the project now focused on medicine and the strategies adopted to ensure continuing independence and authority in the face of demands for greater public accountability. My primary objective was to discover how this profession kept control over its area of expert practice and over the conditions under which that practice could flourish. To take interpretations and understandings beyond one particular sequence of events and extend them to the nature of professions and the processes of professionalization would require the development of valid and comprehensive theory. As the conflict continued, the urgency of understanding what was happening and interpreting the clash of interests and ideologies energized our endeavours. Nonetheless, the chronicle of these events remained secondary. The research was to be directed beyond the specificities of one contest and was to be engaged with more general concerns: the ways by which professions secure their privileged position and take command in matters of birth, death, freedom, justice – those things that lie at the centre of universal human concern.

At the same time it became apparent that the authority of public administration and its different bases of power were equally relevant to theories about what, how and why events turned out as they did. So an examination of the nature of the state, in particular the Australian state, was required. The task now extended to developing an interpretation of the clash of ideologies and cultures as well as the prolonged discord of political and economic interests.

In all research the business of theorizing continues before, throughout and after the empirical enquiries are finished. It is essential to begin with a theoretical perspective, a way of ordering and interpreting what is found. But research is an exploration and theory must be held lightly and discarded or revised according to what is discovered. Sociologists can choose from a number of theories selected for likely applicability to particular conditions as well as for concurrence with the values, opinions and experiences of the researchers themselves.

There is the sphere of meta-theory – grand, overarching, abstract perspectives that make minimal assumptions about the nature of the social context and claim the widest applicability. The modern system builders, from Comte to Giddens or Marx to Habermas operate at this level. The level of abstraction is heady and exciting, like climbing a mountain peak; but bringing meta-theory to bear on particular cases is difficult (as one comes down from the mountain the view gets obstructed).

At a less ambitious level of generality are the middle-level theories that restrict interpretation to cultural, social, political and economic specificities. These theories should hold true across defined places and times. They make no claim for cross-cultural validity or trans-historical persistence. Middle-level theories incorporate parameters such as the political-economic system, the organization of services, the exigencies of the period (such as war, peace, recession). A lot of conceptually sound and practically demonstrable theories are produced at this level of generality.

Grounded theory, as the term denotes, emerges from the data as it is analysed. The data collection and analysis are rigorously systematic and directed to eliciting the general factors and principles that affect the phenomena being studied. More particular and more sensitive to contingencies, grounded theory presumes very little and brings a range of concepts or co-ordinating ideas to the task of organizing subjective accounts and observations.

Preliminary theories are prejudgements (for which one may read 'prejudged' or 'biased') and serve as heuristic devices for ordering the data. It is therefore important that the theoretical perspective which informs research planning and practice should recognize the significant players and encompass the dynamics of the events and processes under study. In the early phases of planning a number of organizing theories may be considered. Our research enterprises are likely to use the sociological theories which we have appropriated over the years. We use what we know already. (Much later, imagination and observation can engender new concepts and theories.) Discipline-based study provides a range of perspectives from which we almost unconsciously draw the conceptual tools needed for research.

Exemplifying this initial theorizing was a review of Marxist perspectives that might have served me well for understanding the dynamics of conflict between two powerful historical blocs, profession and state. One point of view urged that underlying the dispute were the material interests of the dominant class repudiating the growth of welfare, specifically health services, and that the medical profession faction was temporarily out of line with its more general class interests – those being well served by the state's practices for containment. In this view the doctors were acting out of false consciousness and ignoring their real interests. Concomitant with this approach the trade unionists, opposed to the doctors' stand, would seem to have betrayed their class interests. A Marxist interpretation did encapsulate some aspects of the conflict, but it ignored the common class origins of the major parties – doctors, senior public servants and politicians (members of Cabinet) – caught up in angry debate. Equally dubious was the assumption of false consciousness, of blindness to 'real' interests, whose attribution to any group I find incomprehensible and disingenuous. Quite simply I do not believe that any group falls into false consciousness for any significant time. People are not blind to their own material interests. The initially promising Marxist paradigm was rejected because it neither addressed the essential dimensions of the struggle nor allowed a comprehensive interpretation of significant factors.

My inclination towards invoking a Weberian approach to this study of conflicts about authority and material interests came readily from studying Weber's analyses of the dynamics of bureaucracy and the

development of law from a multiplicity of ideal and material influences.
(Theory sensitizes the inquirer to ideas that are potentially significant.)
Weberian concepts germane to sociology and politics were clearly going
to be useful in this research. It was obvious at a very early stage that
the conflict was about 'power and money'; the authority of the state
and the authority of knowledge and skill; the influence of the expert
or the scientist on a field of practice and the regulatory imperatives
guiding the task of the official or bureaucrat; the material interests
of private practitioners and public providers. And there were other
conceptual tools, ways of abstracting and summarizing salient
processes which were applied. Some of these constructs, such as
'corporate culture' of workplace or group, the solidarity of collegiate
and profession, the social constraints encountered by individual action,
owe much to the sociology of Emile Durkheim. Other ways of seeing
and interpreting have become familiar in more recent political and
sociological writing – the processes of agenda setting, mobilization
of forces, sloganeering, courting media partisanship, leverage of
strategic lobbying, promulgation of partial expert opinion, of
delegitimation, exploitation of regulation and law-making pushed to
(and over) the limit. Most significant in the task of theory-building
was a return in late 20th century thinking to a fascination with the
utter contingency of human affairs.

A striking example of the role of contingency in human affairs was
a series of events in a country hospital which shifted negotiations
drastically. Medical services at a large country hospital ceased when
the visiting specialist radiologist withdrew her services and equipment
because of a unilateral alteration of conditions of medical practice in
public hospitals. The shock of this woman's resistance shuddered
through the New South Wales health system and prompted the
withdrawal of the most contentious section of the Government's
regulations. Without pre-empting the more detailed account in *Medicine
and the State* (Daniel, 1990) a series of contingencies significantly shifted
the balance of power. The indeterminacy of individual action can
demolish a too rigid structuralist theory.

This discussion of my attempts at theory-building suggests
instructive aspects of the business of theorizing that can be highlighted.

5. *The theoretical perspective, often called paradigm, from which the
researcher operates is one which will accord with his or her experience
of being human, of being a social being. 'What sort of philosophy (theory)
one chooses depends, therefore, on what sort of person one is; for a philosophical
system is not a dead piece of furniture that we can reject or accept as we wish;
it is rather a thing animated by the soul of the person who holds it'* (Fichte,
1982 [1797]).

6. *The theory to direct the planning of the project should be chosen for its apparent comprehension of and relevance to the institutions, processes and outcomes under study. It should be held lightly as a heuristic device for organizing, ordering and making sense of what is discovered. And it should be reinforced, modified or rejected to ensure that the best interpretation emerges at the end. The 'best' is that which remains true to the research findings, promotes understanding and enables that understanding to be generalized to other times, places and sets of conditions.*

RESEARCH REFINING THEORY

Theory serves to order and organize the research process, interprets what is discovered and goes beyond the contingencies of the particular situation. Theory derives more abstract and generalizable understandings of social action and institutions in fields like those traversed in studying health-related issues. As has been intimated the theory derived from the study of conflict between profession and state was refined and modified as the research continued. While the practical work of the study went on, new books and articles demanded careful and critical scrutiny; these prompted fresh ideas and suggested more constructs useful in the task of developing a comprehensive sociological interpretation. The work of other sociologists focused on medical dominance, particularly Evan Willis in Australia and Paul Starr in the USA, reinforced the persuasiveness of theories of professionalization put forward by Freidson and Rueschemeyer. The interpretation I reached owes much to these sociologists and other more abstract theorists (the structuration theories of Anthony Giddens and the sophisticated general theory of Jeffrey Alexander will be apparent to my critical reader).

In developing theory the researcher often ranges widely and draws ideas and concepts from discourses beyond those concerned with a particular area of study. For instance, although it is not at all concerned with professions or health services, Alexander's synthesizing account of 'action and its environments' (1988) could be most useful in identifying the crucial elements to be addressed in systematic health resarch. There will be found a linking of the 'micro' and 'macro' levels appropriate to reviewing trends and examining events in the health field; the theory encompasses the way individuals interpret and strategically direct their interests within a culturally constructed 'reality'; it recognizes the constant relevance of the constraints on action imposed by structures (for 'culturally constructed reality' the health researcher might read professional or organizational cultures and for 'structure' hospitals or community-based organizations). An excursion into Alexander's very detailed thesis is not called for here.

Rather the empirical researcher is urged to engage with the abstractions and generalizations of sociological theory to raise pertinent issues, guide analysis and inform the interpretation of research findings.

To a considerable extent theory directs which research strategies will be adopted. A diversity of methods are required where the theoretical orientation recognizes the importance of the larger social, political and economic context, the normative, or value-laden culture of workplace or organization and the structural or contingent resistances to individual interests. Here the imagination and resourcefulness of the researcher comes into play. And so comes the next point:

7. Inevitably that preliminary theory, unless it is remarkably abstracted and general, will undergo changes. If nothing unexpected turns up doubt the validity of the enquiry and return to the field. (No theory anticipates everything in human affairs.) The interdependency of theory and research is such that the researcher develops theoretically driven interpretations by moving constantly between 'fact' and 'interpretation', between empirical discovery and sociological theory.

HISTORICALLY INFORMED RESEARCH

Critically relevant to my task in studying the doctors' dispute was an examination of how the contending parties had developed their present political, ideational and material character. All social research, including health research, must be historically informed. Unless we know what came before we cannot understand the present character of the actors and the socially created structures which confront and resist them. It was apparent from the beginning that a careful examination of the history of events and trends that produced the present would be necessary. How else would it be possible to understand the culture of the hospital, or the significance of public hospital appointment? Where else might the origins of critical changes in the management of health services be found? Why was restructuring of large institutions chosen as the response to diminished funds?

Exemplifying the need for investigating history was the problem of explaining the difficulties faced by one of the main parties in the dispute. Morale in the New South Wales State Health Department was low; many of its officers were suffering a sense of anomy, of being without intelligible guidelines, of alienation from their colleagues, from accustomed duties and from the overall policies of their organization. The sources of these discontents became apparent from the recent history of politically driven restructuring, rationalization of key activities and reformulation of management philosophies and objectives. Finding out about all this entailed a perusal of reports produced from commissions and inquiries such as the Coombs Royal Commission, the Review of New South Wales Administration (Wilenski, 1977), the Commission of Inquiry into the Efficiency and Administration of Hospitals. The search continued through newspaper stories of the abolition of the Health Commission and establishment of a Department with limited functions and less autonomy. The enabling legislation gave a more precise and rigid account of this restructuring. The parliamentary record *Hansard* detailed the arguments about significant changes in policy and administrative arrangements.

This experience leads to an important point in this catalogue of research imperatives:

8. Health research requires careful enquiry into the history of organizations and associations that form part of the area under study. To do this the researcher must learn and adopt the basic skills of the historian and utilize all available documents that bear on the character, objectives and expectations of organizations and groups germane to the study. These documents will be directed to purposes different from the researcher's and can be sharply slanted in their accounts. Recognition of some inevitable bias is part of the task of keeping their usefulness within the bounds of validity and reliability.

DISCERNING CULTURE

Nowhere is sensitivity to culture and subculture more important than in health research. To some extent the culture of work organizations and healthcare institutions can be described from their history, but that only brings us to present conditions.

Observations, as a participant or accepted onlooker, is the way to understanding the meanings, values and modes of action that inform the social construction of any association or organization. In health studies the culture of dominant institutions, particularly hospitals, can be described in terms of traditionally grounded values, shared standards and staunch co-operation within the group. Durkheim's model of 'mechanical solidarity' has remarkable application to doctors or nurses at work in public hosptials. If this solidarity is carried over into larger associations and unions it generates a strength reinforced by conflict with other organizations. The imaginative researcher will conjure a number of strategies to allow a close and sustained study of group culture. Many health studies have utilized an opening for a legitimate participant assisting in the work of the place. In my particular study much of the political manoeuvring was planned in meetings and the issues were publicized in protest demonstrations and statements. Public meetings such as Labour Council sessions and demonstrations were readily accessed. I sought and gained permission to attend professional meetings and political briefings. Beyond these more formal occasions was the feeling for the issues that was engendered as we hurried from interview to interview in hospital wards, health departments and the homes of those caught in the conflict. This experience recalls the first point raised in this chapter, the enhanced salience of the social context in times of high stress and sharp conflict. The further point this raises is important:

9. *The cultural context colours the way trends and events are perceived and determines the ambit of possible action. In coming to an understanding of the culture of place and group there is no satisfactory substitute for 'being there', for sociologically perceptive and systematic observation. The sensitizing function of theory has further application in observation studies.*

ASKING QUESTIONS

I have given privileged position to a focus on history and a concern with observation in this critical review of my own research. These laid the basis for an intelligent engagement in long and relatively unstructured interviews with protagonists of all points of view. The questions taken up in interviews were determined by the participant's interests in and views of controversy and conflict. A list of items to be raised served to prompt discussion and ensure that all potential concerns were raised. The list was essential as the interviewing continued over months, sometimes in joint sessions but more often carried out by one of us singly. The need to ensure that interviews could flag all relevant matters for discussion was reinforced when some were conducted by telephone. Obviously these latter lacked the immediacy of communication in person. The productive potential of directed discussion with those involved prompts another proposition:

10. *Face-to-face interviewing of those immediately involved in the events and processes under study should be structured only to the extent necessary to ensure comprehensiveness and comparability. The accounts given and the way these are formulated should be determined by the participant rather than the interviewer. Questionnaires are different. In contrast to the interview they are constructed to give the questioner's agenda priority.*

SAMPLING: PURPOSE AND GENERALITY

Validity, reliability and sound representation are the objectives of good sampling techniques. The objective of the sampling method chosen is always to secure a representative cover of facts, values, opinions, expectations held by those peopling the field of study. The requirement that those asked know about or can be expected to know about the issues raised is an important validity criterion. To ensure that sectional views are represented a variety of techniques are set out in the textbooks.

This study of the medical profession and the state sought out the leaders of all contesting parties. Those leading the medical profession in their battles were identified by their prominence in public debates and the recommendation of those publicly identified as leading and speaking for the medical groups involved. The networking approach to identifying and seeking out the opinion leaders is one commonly used in studies of elites. Officers of the Health Department were not as highly visible, but those most responsible for Health department responses to the crises could be identified by their seniority and their immediate involvement with provision of hospital services and related personnel and industrial problems. In Weberian terms those to be sought for interview were the key position-holders in the health bureaucracy. With this group also, referral by others sent me to officers who held informed and articulate views about the crises developing in the state's hospitals. I had had earlier research contacts in the Department and that, I think, gave some grounds for trusting me with confidences. As with the doctors, a critical factor in allowing an interview was the wish to ensure that their account be eventually presented fairly. It was similarly possible to talk with trade union officials and gain views, both public-spirited and partisan. Consumer-interest leaders were not to the fore in this conflict, although it was clear that patients were suffering badly. A very few were contacted by phone and gave their views on the self-centred blindness of all concerned; it is sad to relate that these fragmented interests had neither the political authority nor the strategic importance to take part in the struggles over medical services in hospitals.

I was able to interview administrators of some major hospitals, but many preferred not to talk personally; their positions were vulnerable and many simply withdrew from engagement with the issues. Politicians could be identified with one of two camps in this complex and cross-cutting conflict. Those in the Government ignored all requests for interviews, although I did receive countless press releases. A very few personal acquaintances in the Government obliged with off-the-record information and explanations. Those in the parliamentary Opposition used the interview for polemical purposes. The book is harsh towards politicians and their draconian invocation of legislation to suit political purposes. Perhaps if I had been allowed near, a more sympathetic understanding of the politicians' dilemma may have emerged.

Is there a guideline for sampling that will be appropriate to research that shares the uncontrollability and unpredictability encountered in this work? The point to be made is:

11. Sampling procedures are always advised by the purpose and intent of the field research. In a study of conflict identify the leaders of the main interest groups and those with whom the leaders confer. Be as open as possible to intimations of where authority or influence lies. Endeavour to speak with all the protagonists. Rarely will that counsel of perfection be possible, so speak with as many as time and resources allow and declare in the report the extent of coverage. A useful sign that the answers are meeting the criterion of representativeness appears when the responses from one group continue to fall readily and repetitively into major categorical patterns.

ETHICAL RESPONSIBILITY

It is paramount in health research to do no harm. This general imperative for all research translates in the health field into a respect for confidentiality and the anonymity of informants and advisers, wherever these are required or advisable. The research into the doctors' dispute was originally focused on discovering how professions dominate and control their field of practice and the character of the interdependence of profession and state which underpins this dominance. Some significant insights emerged. Regardless of my own interests, I owe the participants a fair publication of the understandings that their participation had allowed.

Sociological research is concerned with exploring, discovering and coming to know how and why particular outcomes eventuate. In the light of such understandings the sociologist can readily become an advocate for the people of the research. It is easy to take sides. In the interests of truth (the ideal most recently claimed for critical theory by Habermas) and, more feasibly, in line with giving a fair and persuasive account, the researcher should seek out and consult with all parties in conflict. The advocacy can then be directed away from a narrowly adversorial function and turned towards resolving or abating the strife and reconciling the conflicting interests. Is this another canon of perfection? Perhaps, but one that recognizes the social responsibility of the sociologist to create a more human society. I conclude then with the following point:

12. The researcher should never ignore the obligation to those who give information and advice or who allow her into their own domain to watch the way they live their lives. The reciprocity implicit in this trust constitutes an obligation to be honoured by a sharing of knowledge (reporting back) and a promotion of understanding of the participants' actions and interests. It is good practice to seek out all sides of conflict, so that, when the researcher becomes (inevitably) an advocate, the advocacy will be more balanced and point in some way to more just solutions.

REFERENCES

Alexander, J.G. (1988) *Action and Its Environments: Towards a New Synthesis*, Columbia University Press, New York.

Daniel, Ann (1983) *Power, Privilege and Prestige: Occupations in Australia*, Longman Cheshire, Melbourne.

Daniel, Ann (1990) *Medicine and the State: Professional Autonomy and Public Accountability*, Allen & Unwin, Sydney.

Fichte, J.G. (1982 [1797]) *Science of Knowledge* (ed. and trans. P. Heath and J. Lachs), Cambridge University Press, Cambridge.

Freidson, Eliot (1986) *Professional Powers: A Study of the Institutionalization of Formal Knowledge*, University of Chicago Press, Chicago.

Rueschemeyer, D. (1986) *Power and the Division of Labour*, Polity Press, Cambridge.

Starr, Paul (1982) *The Social Transformation of American Medicine*, Basic Books, New York.

Willis, Evan (1983) *Medical Dominance: The Division of Labour in Australian Health Care*, Allen & Unwin, Sydney.

CHAPTER 2

Methodological and political issues in occupational health research

Michael Gliksman

INTRODUCTION

Occupational health research provides unique challenges which encompass political as well as methodological considerations. Problems related to the formulation and conduct of epidemiological health research in an industrial setting are largely political in nature. It follows that a satisfactory solution is dependent on an appreciation of the politics involved.

Whilst disagreement and controversy are no strangers to any aspect of health research, the often adversorial and at times acrimonious nature of union/management relations means these often feature most prominently in occupational health research. Unless overcome, this may seriously affect the ability to carry out scientifically valid studies in such settings. When initial reluctance by a multinational employer to undertake research to address the health and safety concerns of a section of its workforce meets the 'gung-ho' approach of trade union health and safety organizers, the main losers are likely to be the workers themselves. How can employer groups be convinced that it is in their interests to discover whether industrial processes and work practices are injurious to the health of their employees? How can the mutual distrust between unions and employers which serves to compromise the ability to perform valid epidemiological research be minimized? What research designs are best suited to this environment? Further, the nature of the questions asked in these settings and the need for results with minimum delays, due to both industrial pressures and the need to minimize continuing harm, often limit the choice of research designs which can be used. This chapter outlines an actual case study in an industrial setting which illustrates these problems and discusses their resolution.

I will first discuss the problems, which had two main aspects, to arise from the research into the potential for manganese-induced neurotoxicity amongst miners, that forms the basis of this chapter. The first problem was the mineworkers' unresolved concern about possible damage to their health. The second was the conflict between the multinational company and the unions regarding the need for and the methods to be employed in any investigation of these concerns. I will then detail the suggestions that became part of the successful resolution of these problems. These include the need for a literature review, an independent management structure, consideration of the advantages and disadvantages of available study designs, and the need for confidentiality.

THE PROBLEMS

Over the years, evidence had been accumulating, primarily from Third World countries, that miners exposed to manganese dusts in high concentrations could suffer from irreversible central nervous system (CNS) damage. The symptoms and signs indicated damage primarily to the basal ganglia which was similar to that found in Parkinson's disease but sometimes accompanied by psychosis, and became known as **manganism** (Rom, 1983). Once established, they were not thought to be reversible.

It was also known that at lower levels of exposure, more ephemeral symptoms and signs of neuropsychological damage could occur. These included asthenia, anorexia, apathy, headache, impotence, leg cramps, speech disturbance and memory loss (Braunwald, 1987). These were thought reversible if exposure ceased.

What was not known was the 'safe' level of exposure at which no evidence of damage could be found. Recently however, a well conducted study suggested this level might be quite low – lower than had been thought likely (Roels *et al.*, 1987). This research was conducted in a manganese smelting factory, so exposure was to fume, not dust. Fume, being highly respirable, is likely to be more damaging than dust at a given concentration (Parkes, 1982). Therefore, the relevance of this finding to exposure in miners was unclear.

A large multinational company operates one of the world's largest open-cut manganese mines. A number of measures by that company had been incorporated over the years to minimize exposure, including provision of sealed, air conditioned cabins for machine operators and constant wetting of tailings and roadways. Dust monitoring, carried out over several years, showed exposure to dust was at least one order of magnitude below that known to cause manganism. Nonetheless, as knowledge of the existence of this disease and the potential for damage at lower levels of exposure became widespread, concern among workers became marked. Could the company assure them that no damage was being done to their health?

The initial attempts by the company to answer this question consisted primarily of restating the position that manganism was not known to occur at the levels of exposure encountered at the mine, and no cases of manganism had been recorded among workers at this open cut mine. This response however, did not fully address concerns about more subtle neuropsychological damage at lower levels of exposure. The failure of the company to adequately address this concern led to the first problem. An open field was created for union health and research employees who, ignorant of epidemiology and research methodology, proposed scientifically unsound investigations to answer the workers' concerns. Resistance by the company to such unsound studies was interpreted by the unions and workers as evidence of 'stalling' and of there being 'something to hide'. A stalemate was reached and the threat of widespread industrial action became real.

The issue for me, a medical epidemiologist employed by the multinational company, became how to steer a course through powerful and therefore hazardous interest groups and keep the research valid.

A SOLUTION

The literature review

Often the first question in need of resolution in any field of preventive ˙health is whether concerns can be adequately addressed by the current level of knowledge. Hence the first task in resolving this problem was to undertake a thorough literature review. This revealed that concerns could not be adequately addressed by the current state of knowledge, for reasons already presented. The effect of this finding in helping galvanize action was dramatic, for several reasons.

First, as the literature review was carried out by an employee from within the company, senior management was more likely to accept its conclusions. It therefore became difficult for the company to resist further investigations into the workers' concerns and prepared the ground for the establishment of a definitive research project. Second, it was then possible to demonstrate to senior management that the long-term costs of inaction were likely to far outweigh the short-term costs of even a large-scale epidemiologically sound study. Third, it suggested to the unions, and the workers they represented, that the company might be willing to deal with the concerns expressed in a manner capable of resolving them.

The management committee

As a consensus developed between the unions and management as to the need for a study, a second problem emerged. The union health and safety representatives wished to determine the methodology to be used and in particular, the personnel utilized to supervise, carry out and analyse the study. Not surprisingly this was deemed unacceptable by the company, which would be funding the study. The counter suggestion that the company appoint personnel from within its ranks to conduct the study, including myself, was equally unacceptable to the unions. Again, an impasse common to the field of occupational health research was reached.

I proposed a possible resolution which was accepted by all parties involved. My proposal included the setting up of an independent management committee to oversee the development and conduct of the research project. The committee was to comprise university academics at professorial level from disciplines relevant to the study's subject. The unions and company management were to provide nominees and appointments would be made from those acceptable to both parties.

The final composition of the committee included the company's Director of Occupational and Environmental Health and Safety, the union's peak body Health and Safety Officer, an emeritus professor of psychology, a professor of biostatistics and an associate professor of clinical epidemiology. The latter assumed overall supervisory responsibility for the study's design and execution. I was commissioned by the management committee to design and write the principles and detailed protocol for the study. The protocol was then to be approved by the committee and selected overseas experts prior to its implementation. This last step was essential in assuring all parties of the adequacy of the final study protocol.

The protocol

The circumstances that would have rendered a protocol developed by a company employee unacceptable to the unions had been negated by the measures already outlined. Therefore, methodological and ethical considerations were able to dominate the protocol developmental process.

In any field of health research results are desired as quickly and as inexpensively as possible. This leads to an understandable drive towards cross-sectional or retrospective research designs when prospective designs, especially randomized controlled trials (Fletcher, Fletcher and Wagner, 1988) may yield more valid results in the long run. It is difficult however, to imagine an industrial situation in which a randomized controlled trial could be ethically acceptable. Assigning groups of workers (randomly or otherwise) to different levels of exposure to a substance or process hypothesized to be injurious to their health and awaiting the outcome clearly could not be justified. Further, in the case of certain disease processes (especially cancers), several decades may elapse between exposure and the development of overt disease. Changing standards and work practices may also mean current exposures do not reflect past exposures.

For all these reasons, it is rare for prospective studies to be utilized in occupational health research. When coupled with industrial relations pressures for rapid results, retrospective studies are usually deemed necessary. Despite their potential shortcomings which include the fact that the risk or incidence of disease usually cannot be measured directly (Fletcher, Fletcher and Wagner, 1988), care in their design and execution may make them capable of yielding valid results.

The precise design that can be used will be largely determined by the type and quality of information that is available or that can be gathered. The fundamental requirements for any research is an index of exposure and of outcome, and the ability to test whether one is associated with the other. If any of these elements are lacking, no meaningful research can be undertaken. The two main types of retrospective research design are the case–control and the historical cohort studies. The former is comprised of people who have the disease or outcome of interest plus a group of otherwise similar people who do not have the disease. The researcher then looks backward in time to assess the frequency and degree of exposure to the putative causal agent in both groups. A subset of this study type is a nested case–control study, where cases and controls are drawn from a predefined population. This strategy can minimize bias and improve validity.

In a cohort study, a group of exposed and a group of unexposed persons (a cohort) is followed over time to see what proportion in each group develops the outcome of interest. These proportions can be compared and the effects of exposure on the risk of developing the outcome quantified. As can be seen, this design proceeds forward in time (i.e., it is prospective). The variant of interest here is the historical cohort study. If exposure status (of the cohort assembled in the present time) can be determined from past records, the cohort can be followed forward from those past records and disease status assessed in the present time. Therefore, the historical cohort study is retrospective in nature but simulates a prospective design and can be used to generate incidence data.

Both the case–control and historical cohort studies depend on an ability to assess past exposure in the present time. Where this is not possible, a prevalence (cross-sectional) study becomes the only alternative. In such a study, outcome and exposure are measured as the same point in time. The major disadvantage of this study type is that it is particularly weak in establishing causality. This is because it cannot provide evidence linking preceding exposure to outcomes (for more detailed information on study design types see Fletcher, Fletcher and Wagner, 1988).

All these study types were considered for the study on manganese neurotoxicity. For several years as part of its routine occupational health and safety practice, the company had been collecting data on workers' personal exposure to manganese dust. Hence, good quality exposure data existed which allowed the construction of an index of exposure based on each worker's job description and worksite over time at the mine. As a result, a prevalence study could be eliminated from consideration for the study design.

Since there were no cases of manganism known to exist among miners, a case–control study was irrelevant. Consequently, the historical cohort design was chosen for the study protocol.

Two further important points required resolution before the protocol could be finalized. First, confidentiality had be to ensured for all participants. A particular concern of the mine workers was that if neuropsychological 'problems' were found, what would be the effect on their employment? Conversely, there was the legislative obligation of the company to provide a safe and healthy work environment. This could conceivably include not allowing an impaired worker to operate potentially dangerous machinery which would represent a hazard to work colleagues. Resolution of this conflict included the use of study numbers and not names on all results, the code for which could only be accessed by management committee members.

No individual's results were to be made available to management or the unions except where results indicated impairment significant enough to represent a potential health and safety hazard. In this case all parties (union, company, individual) would be notified and the company undertook to retain the employee in an appropriate position with no loss of pay, seniority or job security. Any other unusual test results would be notified only to the individual and his or her medical adviser under a confidentiality agreement. Combined with frequent discussions and involvement of on-site worker representatives this measure ensured a good participation rate which was essential to the validity of the study.

Second, as in any field of health research, it was essential to ensure that any beliefs relating to the hypothesis of manganese-induced damage held by the research workers were incapable of biasing the results. This was especially important in relation to those administering the neuropsychological tests to the mine workers, who were believed by some to hold strong views as to causality.

This was achieved by ensuring that all data collectors/testers were unaware of the exposure status of the worker (this is known as 'blinding') being tested. Hence it was not possible for the testers to (consciously or unconsciously) bias the test results. It was only at the point of statistical analysis of all results that exposure data, which was collected separately from all other data, was cross-linked to the results of individual testing.

CONCLUSIONS

While not all research activities in occupational medicine may overcome the very considerable political and industrial impediments they may meet, it should be clear from the foregoing case summary that adherence to certain principles can smooth the path and maximize the chances of a professionally satisfying and scientifically valid conclusion.

First and foremost among these is to avoid the temptation to tell employers what they want to hear. Instead, tell them what they should hear. Whilst the alternative approach may seem at times expedient, it represents an abrogation of professional responsibilities and is likely to have its consequences. The principle of 'garbage in–garbage out' applies; inadequate advice will lead to poor decisions which may eventually cost the workers their health and the company lost production and profits, not to mention the potential for legal action. Ultimately, as the 'expert', responsibility for the consequences will track back to you.

Second, bland assurances such as 'there's never been a problem before' are often misleading and always inadequate. Early action to investigate health and welfare concerns is essential. This may need to be no more than an adequate literature review or, as previously described, a full scale epidemiological study. Failure to take early action invites mistrust and leaves an 'open field' for charlatans and the ignorant to force the pace and undermine the potential for a scientifically credible investigation.

Third, a management committee comprised of experts independent of unions and management is needed to oversee the development of any study protocol, the conduct of the study and the analysis of the resultant data. This ensures that not only will an unbiased investigation be carried out, it will be seen to be unbiased by all parties. This in turn makes it far more likely that the conclusions will be accepted by all parties and acted upon.

Fourth, assurances to the workforce of confidentiality of individual results and guarantees that no negative consequences will occur based on those individual results is essential if co-operation and a good participation rate are expected.

Fifth, in order to minimize the risk of bias, those responsible for gathering outcome data should be unaware of each participant's exposure status. This safeguard may be strengthened by separating the tasks of exposure and outcome data gathering, and data analysis.

Last but definitely not least, whilst design is usually a compromise reflecting ethical as well as scientific realities, everything is negotiable except the scientific validity of the study. Compromise that and the workers will be the ultimate losers.

REFERENCES

Braunwald, E. (1987) *Harrison's Principles of Internal Medicine*, 11th edn, McGraw-Hill, New York.

Fletcher, R.H., Fletcher, S.W. and Wagner, E.H. (1988) *Clinical Epidemiology – the Essentials*, 2nd edn, Williams & Wilkins, Baltimore.

Parkes, W.R. (1982) *Occupational Lung Disorders*, 2nd edn, Butterworth & Co, London.

Roels, H., Lauwerys, R. and Buchet, J.P. *et al.* (1987) Epidemiological survey among workers exposed to manganese: effects on lung, central nervous system, and some biological indices. *Am. J. Ind. Med*, **11** (3), 307–27.

Rom, W.N. (1983) *Environmental and Occupational Medicine*, Little, Brown & Company, Boston.

CHAPTER 3

Team research in clinical settings: strategies for the qualitative researcher

Jeanne Daly

INTRODUCTION

A team is a group drawn together for a common purpose, a purpose which the individual cannot achieve alone. Individual action is necessarily constrained. A team of draught oxen is yoked and bound, and even whipped, so that they pull in one direction. Teams of people are more commonly directed by rules which define the role of each team member and place limits on what the individual may do. Learning to play a team game requires the development of individual skills and learning the rules of the game.

Sometimes the rules of a game are well established and inflexible. A game is played on a field of given dimensions and goals are scored, say, between set goal posts. Sometimes, especially if a game is new, the rules are flexible and negotiable. Australian Rules football, for example, was first played in open city parkland (Blainey, 1990). Captains decided before a match where the goal posts would be. Trees were accepted obstacles and when the ball got stuck up a tree, or was deflected off a tree trunk, teams improvised. The idiosyncratic rules for the Australian game developed over time to reflect local conditions.

The multidisciplinary research teams of this chapter involve clinicians and sociologists. Since this research game is relatively new, rules are unclear and obstacles abound which make the flow of the game unpredictable. My aim is not to specify rules for multidisciplinary research but to discuss the negotiating process for changing the rules of clinical research so that sociologists can contribute their special skills. Sociologists are the suppliants – like short basketball players who are pressuring the League to change the rules so that they may participate without disadvantage. They have to present their case persuasively.

In the first section I set out the reasons why it is worthwhile negotiating team research instead of 'going it alone'. The first step is to negotiate goals so that the research is of benefit to both sociologists and clinicians. I then discuss negotiating the rules of the game, developing agreement about what is to count as good research without compromising the essentials of sociological method. I deal with each step of the research process in turn: entering the field, selecting a sample, analysing the data and ensuring validity and generalizability. The outcome of the research should contribute to both sociological and medical knowledge. It should also contribute to an increased understanding of research method in general and the methods appropriate for multidisciplinary work.

MULTIDISCIPLINARY TEAMS

Clinical practice is a rich area of research for sociologists since the social context is of central importance but substantially under-researched. Doctors come from particular social backgrounds, train in medical institutions and enter medical practice in the private or public sphere. We do not yet understand how this social context influences their decision making, including what they say and do with patients. Consultations, the central event in medical care, are social interactions with patients who come from different social backgrounds which influence what they say in the consultation, and how they come to understand it later, at home. Advice from family, friends and media reports may further mediate both patient understanding and compliance with medical advice. This effects health outcome but we know little about what the outcome is or what its main determinants are.

Consultations often involve technical matters like prescribing a drug or ordering a test. Sociologists seldom have the technical knowledge necessary for analysing these procedures. If they misrepresent technical or biomedical fact it discredits their research in the eyes of medical colleagues. Clinicians, on the other hand, seldom have the specialist sociological skill required for analysing the social context. The self-evident solution is to bring the two complementary sets of skills together in a multidisciplinary team.

There is a lack of good sociological analysis of medical care from multidisciplinary teams. This may be because physicians see the critical attitudes of sociology as mere 'doctor bashing' – and they are the gatekeepers to access. A more important problem may well be that they do not understand sociological research methods, with qualitative method heading the list. Sociologists may also take for granted their own assumptions of what counts as good research. Thus the potential for misunderstanding is high and discussions of method are often surprisingly contentious. The advantage is that it forces researchers from both disciplines to re-examine their own basic assumptions about research methodology in order to reach the best possible resolution of differences.

As in most team activities there are some obvious ways in which team work can be improved. Team members need agreement on a common goal and the rules of the game. These need to be argued through on a point-by-point basis. There should be a clear and acceptable role for all members of the team. It is important that sociologists should not be seen as the mere handmaidens of clinician-researchers but the concerns of clinicians need to be addressed in a constructive manner. A more difficult issue for clinicians may be the argument that the consumers of healthcare, patients, also need a voice, that their views have the same legitimacy as those of clinicians or sociologists.

What I intend to cover in this contribution are the ways in which I, as a qualitative researcher, have negotiated research in clinical settings with medical co-researchers. An important obstacle is often the emphasis which sociologists put on the use of theory. I take it for granted that this is a necessary part of sociological skill but, in this context, some of it may need to be thought through by the sociologist in private. I concentrate here on the public negotiations aimed at ensuring that the research process does not unnecessarily compromise the very real strengths of a long-established sociological tradition of research. What follows is a recounting of common issues and possible ways of constructive resolution.

DEFINING THE GOAL

The goal for multidisciplinary research often arises from the concerns of practitioners although the original concern may have been raised by policy makers. Since the 1970s, for example, policy makers have been concerned about the proliferation of expensive medical tests. An increasingly important use of tests is to reassure anxious patients that they are normal, and using tests in this way can lead to escalating medical costs. Clinicians, on the other hand, worry that patients reassured by a negative test result may not remain reassured in the longer term.

What is sometimes less evident is that the research must also address a question which has sociological significance. Sociologists are not lone operators. Our methods depend upon locating research within the body of theoretical and empirical sociological research. Our aim is to apply what we know about social life to a particular context so that we add to our body of knowledge by extending what we know or resolving contradictions. The literature gives us our sense of problem and our results must be coherent with it.

We need to distinguish between research which merely addresses social problems and sociological research. A social problem might well be to find out whether a negative test result more effectively reassures working class or middle class patients, men or women. Sociologists might find a 'handmaiden' role in devising measures for these social categories but a more sociological goal would be to draw on what we know about class, medical institutions, communication and culture to explain why some groups of patients are not reassured. Another example of a social problem might be to identify which teenagers do not practice safe sex so that information-giving can be effectively targetted. The sociologically significant problem might be to understand the social and sexual relations of groups of teenagers, including social barriers to young girls initiating condom usage.

Defining the question for research requires negotiation with co-researchers so that the research addresses the practitioners' practical concerns and is of sociological significance. Often this involves difficult negotiations about who are the proper 'objects' of the research. Clinicians tend to locate problems in the behaviour of patients and focus study on these alone. This may mean, as happened recently, that typists transcribing tapes of consultations are instructed to leave out what the doctor says, only transcribing patient responses.

More recently there has been medical acknowledgement of the importance of doctor–patient communication. This makes it easier to argue for the taping and full transcription of consultations. The pre-occupation of clinicians, however, is with controlling a clinical event and any aspects of a study which do not contribute to this goal may be seen as irrelevant to the study. An example follows.

My first study in a clincial setting evaluated the effectiveness of a normal text result from echocardiography (cardiac ultrasound) in reassuring patients that their hearts are normal (Daly, 1989). The cardiologists were concerned to know why reassurance fails. They believed that patients who are not reassured either forget what they are told or have a neurotic investment in being ill. This hypothesis could be tested by measuring patients' anxiety before and after a normal test result and then testing for recall and neuroses. This conceptualization was too limited even from a medical perspective: if the hypothesis were confirmed, it would tell us little about why it should be so and what to do about it. From a sociological per-spective, the consultation following a test is best seen not as an isolated clinical event controlled by the doctor, but as a social process with potential problems arising at any point along the way. We needed to know more about the social context of both cardiologists and patients. We needed to know what 'reassurance' means in the medical culture, why the test was ordered and how the test result was used in the consultation. We needed to know how patients came to be referred for the test, how they responded to referral and what part they took in the consultation. Finally we needed to know how patients made sense of their experience later. The consultation is therefore the intersecting node of two very different social contexts.

There was some resistance from the cardiologists to this more complex formulation of the problem. It required that they admit their own activities as a proper 'object' of study. But the broader focus for the study had a better chance of addressing their own major concern, understanding why reassurance fails.

These negotiations took over six months but it was not time wasted. During this time I discussed the research process with other cardiologists who had worked with sociologist-researchers. In one unit they were concerned about difficulties in communicating with seriously ill cardiac patients. They were very angry about a sociologist who had done research in the unit and 'exploited' them, debating sociological problems in language they did not understand and leaving them no better off in coping with their problems. They rejected the findings; in fact they could not understand them. In contrast, our aim was to ensure that practitioners' problems were directly addressed (if not resolved), and that they would learn something about their practice, thus improving access for subsequent sociologists. A common commitment to the research would, we hoped, sustain the team during the frustrations which occur during most research projects. It should also mean that policy recommendations would be more acceptable.

Having decided on the goal, the next stage is to define the rules of the game by addressing issues of method. The most common concern of medical co-researchers is that sociological method, especially qualitative method, is not constrained by what they recognize as the rules of scientific research.

NEGOTIATING THE RULES OF THE GAME

Negotiating the rules of the research game with clinicians is slow, comparable with trying to persuade a basketball league that players should be allowed to kick the ball. It requires a talking through of possible positive and negative implications of changing the rules.

Similarities and differences between the methods which clinicians understand best and qualitative method need to be clarified. Here I rehearse the kinds of arguments which I have found useful.

Underlying qualitative sociological research and medical research are the same scientific concerns: to develop ways of structuring the collection and analyis of data so that the results are scientifically valid. There are two different ways of going about it, much simplified here. We need to choose which is the appropriate set of rules for the particular research problem.

Quantitative research is more appropriate when the problem involves a limited set of variables. There may be a validated research instrument for measuring variables. Data represent objective measures of what happens and they aim to be free of the values of both the 'objects' of research and the researchers. In this way data are stripped of their context so that comparisons can be made of what different people do in different situations. With a limited number of variables, data can be collected from a larger number of units (the sample). This allows statistical control over bias and chance error, and increases the generalizability of the results. In the classic experiment the number of variables is statistically further reduced so that the result is expressed as a cause and effect. The internal validity of the study depends upon the rigour of the statistical analysis of the data and the external validity depends upon how representative the sample is of the population from which it was drawn.

Qualitative research is much more difficult to define – like the rules you would need for a game where the playing field is covered in fog and you cannot see either boundaries or goalposts. The rules of the game must be flexible enough to allow research to happen, but not undisciplined. Since researchers cannot prespecify or limit the number of relevant variables for data collection, they have to collect unstructured 'slices of life' – any data relevant to the research question. Data often concern the dynamics of a social setting, are context-dependent and can include documents, observation and tape recorded interviews. It all depends on what we find when we get there. The data collected are extensive, so the number of units from which the data are drawn (the 'sample', for want of a better word) is often small.

Data analysis consists of structuring and condensing the full range of data for analysis. If we do not know in advance what the data are going to be, we cannot say exactly how to analyse it. The analysis itself is presented in the form of an argument explaining what has been observed and relating it to the research question. The internal validity of the study rests on the convincing nature of the argument, its capacity to account for the full variety of data and to make a case for the conclusions (Silverman, 1989). If a study is coherent with the body of existing knowledge, if it explains a little more about what we already know and if any differences are argued through convincingly, it gives credibility to the research, indicating the extent to which its results can be generalized to other **comparable** contexts.

For co-researchers, the emphasis which sociologists place on theory can be confusing. It is worth emphasizing that all disciplines even physics, biomedicine and statistics draw their concepts from theory although this theory is seldom explicitly acknowledged. The coherence with existing theory is also an important way in which we distinguish good research from bad in any discipline. A further difficulty is that the analysis is presented in words, in a reasoned argument, and not merely in statistical symbols. Here it is worth remembering that it is the **logic** of an argument which determines its truth value and not whether this argument is expressed in symbols or words.

Qualitative research is flexibly disciplined: the limits are set by theory and by the situation which we are analysing. Despite such assurances my cardiologist co-researchers still viewed qualitative methods with suspicion. They argued, quite correctly, that a qualitative proposal was less likely to be funded by medically dominated funding bodies and that the conclusions would be less likely to be published by medical journals. They preferred quantitative methods with validated research instruments and larger samples. Unfortunately the problem is not that simple: the choice of research method is not an arbitrary one, dependant on political convenience. As a general rule, quantitative methods are best if we have valid measures of variables which can be abstracted from their context. If testing patients were to be seen as a social process, data would necessarily be context-dependent. Fortunately, one year later, a qualitative research proposal, meticulously justifying the choice of method, passed the funding hurdle.

I now turn to a more detailed look at the different stages of qualitative research.

Entering the field

Qualitative sociologists draw on social anthropology for techniques for entering the field to collect data. The researcher inevitably has some tentative hypotheses based on sociological theory and medical co-researchers may draw on their own knowledge or experience. These set the initial direction for data collection. The overall aim is usually to explain how the study participants see things.

Many qualitative researchers require permission to become passive observers, to blend into the background so that they can unobtrusively gather data on the everyday activities of a setting. This takes time which one often does not want to 'waste' at the start of a project but, in the long term, data collected in this way has an authenticity recognized by the participants. Clinicians are at home in clinical settings and may underestimate problems of entry for sociologists. In my experience, sociologists observing in a hospital or clinical practice need to be as careful to avoid giving offence as anthropologists studying bloodthirsty warriors on the warpath. The problem is most acute where the tension levels are highest, in operating theatres or intensive care, and here projects need to be introduced with exquisite care. I sometimes even explain how I am going to dress in order to avoid being mistaken for a health professional. The alternative of donning a white coat and a stethoscope has been suggested but that misrepresents my role and carries the danger that patients will only tell me what they see as medically acceptable.

Medical co-researchers may fear that sociologists will be 'captured' by factions or special interest groups. Indeed, a structured survey instrument may present as a good way of limiting data to medically acceptable questions, excluding those which might raise uncomfortable issues. The aim of the qualitative researcher, it should be made clear, is not to be judgemental – we do not start by judging who is pushing a barrow, telling the truth or doing a good job, allowing this to influence data collection. Instead we carefully document all differences in attitude. This evidence is then available for all co-researchers to interpret and analyse, at which stage the values of researchers themselves become further 'objects' for analysis.

Theoretical sampling

In medical research samples are often randomly selected. They may feel it necessary to delay analysis until all data have been collected so that early results do not subtly bias later sample selection. To their horror they find that qualitative researchers purposefully select participants based on early analysis of data. This requires careful justification.

The first data are collected from whatever source seems most appropriate for the question. There will be some initial hypotheses but a close reading of the data will generate classifications or categories suggesting additional hypotheses. These hypotheses are tested by searching for supporting or contradictory evidence in the data. This suggests further directions for the collection of data, indicating the need to diversify the sample and the direction that this should take. Hypotheses continue to be generated from and tested in the data as it accumulates and diversifies. This process of gradually developing and refining both hypotheses and supporting evidence is what is meant by 'grounding' theory in data (Strauss, 1987).

Additional categories for classification may come from reading the sociological literature, and medical co-researchers can contribute their own more technical reasons for extending the sample in a particular direction. When the researchers feel confident that they fully understand what is going on, the sample is seen as saturated and data collection ceases. Sample selection for qualitative studies is theoretically disciplined (Strauss, 1987), not based on researcher bias.

Here it is worth explaining that these research processes are comparable with the way in which clinicians take patient histories, flexibly drawing on medical knowledge and clinical training to understand the patient experience.

Analysing the data

The researcher searches through what may be a large volume of data, structuring it into theoretically useful categories. This is not an impressionistic exercise. If, for example, we want to see how patients respond to doctors with different consultation styles, the data may suggest a classification of authoritative or participatory. When categorizing the data in this way we need to define the grounds on which we make this judgement (what is said, in what manner). In a transcript, we need to identify which lines of text support the classification and which suggest a different interpretation. The analysis then takes the form of an argument which explains convincingly how and why patient responses relate to consultation style. In this argument we must account for all supporting and deviant cases; we may draw on other data from the study and we would usually use relevant sociological theory.

Sociologists faced with sceptical colleagues can sometimes lose confidence in their own methods and worry that another researcher might come to a different conclusion. Here it may help to test interpretations more carefully by fully debating the criteria for judging particular categories. In the literature there are usually similar studies and they provide comparisons for the critical assessment of method in the present study. We are not alone in the field but part of a discipline which provides support for what we are doing.

In the echocardiography study, because of the scepticism of the cardiologists, we went further. We drew up a list of 107 categories for grading. So, for example, we were interested in the extent to which doctors in a consultation explained the implications of the test result to the patient. Using a previous study as an example (Tuckett *et al.*, 1985), we devised criteria for what would count as explanation and what would count as high, medium and low levels of explanation.

One of the cardiologists and I graded all the transcripts independently for the 107 variables. We recorded the grading and lines of text supporting the grading on a database. Despite the difference in disciplinary background, statistical tests of interobserver variability were not significant. Often we listed the same lines of text as the basis for a grading. Where gradings differed, we returned to the full transcript to look at what the data said. We were able to agree on the better grading in all but a few cases. This process was time-consuming but it left everyone confident that our data were unbiased, that is 'hard'.

Ensuring validity and generalizability

The internal validity of a study derives from the careful, stepwise, logical unfolding of an argument, accounting for all data and quoting extracts from data where appropriate.

Sociological study, however, gives study participants a special role in research. Some researchers use a format where the researchers and the study participants co-operatively set the directions of the study and generate its conclusions. In more traditional research, an important test of validity is to take the analysis back to the participants for verification. The participants should recognize the study as authentic, and that the researchers have faithfully represented their concerns. Here it is worth emphasizing that this rule applies equally to clinician co-researchers and to patients who participated in the study. Either group may disagree with the conclusions. So, for example, because policy makers, doctors and patients may all hold different views the conclusions of a study may not completely reflect the interests of any of them. Such disagreements must be explained and researchers should also recognize which of their own preconceptions constitute a potential bias.

In order to establish external validity, the study is located within the wider sociological literature, so that the claims which the study makes can be assessed against the body of existing theoretical and empirical work. These claims have to be argued and evidence must be quoted which is sufficiently powerful for us to see the need to accommodate the new claims. Where appropriate the same can be done for the medical literature.

THE OUTCOME OF THE RESEARCH

When playing any game, it is important to know how the game is to be won. With the precautions I have mentioned, the research

should address the sociologist's theoretical and the clinicians's practical interests. In the echocardiography study, presenting the material
to groups of cardiologists drew a positive response: it corresponded
with their experience, setting out clearly the dilemmas of this area
of clinical practice. They saw it as useful in defining potential pitfalls.
This counts as a win.

Qualitative methods are more troublesome when it comes to the
other test: whether the research can be published to inform the clinical
community. Most medical journals set strict limits on the length of
papers and this is a problem given the discursive nature of qualitative
analysis. Three years after submission to a sociological journal (Daly,
1989), this research has been presented at a multidisciplinary conference on research method (Daly *et al.*, 1992), but the cardiologists
have not yet found a satisfactory way of presenting the material for
medical publication. This counts as a loss.

The conclusion of sociological research may sometimes be
unwelcome because it provides a complex answer where a simple one
is sought. Sociological analysis often classifies groups of people
according to their common experience in order to explain why it
happens. One study focused on the relative benefit of surgery and
a non-invasive out-patient procedure (lithotripsy) for the treatment
of gallstones. Qualitative analysis showed that some groups of
patients prefer surgery and some prefer lithotripsy; this choice is
perfectly rational from the patient's point of view. Moreover, one group
of patients did very badly on lithotripsy and another group did very
well. While the average patient experience is about the same for both
procedures, it seemed less significant than recognizing that the benefits
are not evenly distributed across all patients. Policy makers, however,
wanted grounds for funding one procedure or the other, and viewed
with suspicion an outcome which complicated rather than simplified
their decision making. The aim of the evaluation is now being
renegotiated. We should really be helping clinicians decide which
patients will benefit most from surgery and which will benefit from
lithotripsy. Both procedures have value. Focusing on the average
experience may simplify policy options but it will be at the expense
of individual patients. This example illustrates the problem of not
negotiating the research question thoroughly at the beginning but we
had not foreseen the results. This project may well turn out to be a
substantial loss for qualitative method.

CONCLUSION

Doing multidisciplinary research, I have argued, requires constant
negotiation and compromise. To relegate sociologists to the hand-

maiden role is to under-utilize their skills. Research which addresses only sociological concerns will lack relevance to clinicians in their practices. The best compromise is one which recognizes both clinical relevance and sociological significance.

As a general rule, in deciding on research method, we need to define the question that we are addressing clearly and identify the constraints that exist in our area of study. The most important of these is what we already know about an area. The other is what time and resources we have available and the nature of the people who are likely to be the respondents. Within these constraints we then have to choose the study design which will best allow us to address the research questions. In this scheme there is no place for the researcher who blindly applies a favoured method (usually quantitative). If the better method of research is qualitative, negotiations have to be conducted with care. In my account of the negotiation process I have emphasized only the arguments which sociologists should use. What I have not done is to argue for the clinician but this is not to deny that they will have to present their concerns as carefully as sociologists need to do. It is, however, true that clinicians are in the more powerful position and the sociologist has to be more persuasive as a result. The positive effect for both disciplines is that the assumptions of our theory and research method have to be debated and critically re-examined. In the process we learn to distinguish between those aspects of our method that are of central significance and those that we can do without if necessary.

Some of what I have described must sound like a true occupation for masochists. However, if the goal of sociological research is finally to change practice, then the increased relevance of carefully negotiated multidisciplinary research must surely make the pain worthwhile.

REFERENCES

Blainey, G. (1990) *A Game of our Own: The Origins of Australian Football*, Information Australia, Melbourne.

Daly, J. (1989) Innocent murmurs: echocardiography and the diagnosis of cardiac normality. *Sociology of Health and Illness*, 11, (2), pp. 99–116.

Daly, J., McDonald, I., and Willis, E. (1992) Why don't you ask them ... : A qualitative research framework for investigating the diagnosis of cardiac normality, in *Researching Health Care: Designs, Dilemmas and Disciplines*, (eds J. Daly, I. McDonald and E. Willis), Routledge, London, pp. 189–206.

Silverman, D. (1989) Telling convincing stories: a plea for cautious positivism in case-studies, in *The Qualitative-Quantitative Distinction in the Social*

Sciences, (eds B. Glasner and J.D. Moreno), Kluwer Academic Publishers, Dordrecht, pp. 57–77.

Strauss, Anselm L. (1987) *Qualitative Analysis for Social Scientists*, Cambridge University Press, Cambridge.

Tuckett, D., Boulton, M., Olson, C. and Williams, A. (1985) *Meetings Between Experts: An Approach to Sharing Ideas in Medical Consultations*, Tavistock Publications, London.

CHAPTER 4

Teaching health research: social sciences in a physical sciences curriculum

Chris Peterson

INTRODUCTION

This chapter is quite different to the others in this book. They all consist of discussions about methodologies that are appropriate to social sciences research into health related areas. This chapter is unique because it considers social sciences research methodologies appropriate in a teaching curriculum to a physical sciences-based health research training programme at an Australian University of Technology. As such, I raise issues in relation to teaching qualitative and quantitative methods within a 'hard' sciences curriculum that may provide a useful basis for reflection for many of the social scientists who teach within medical, applied health sciences and related courses. I do not intend to be an apologist for the methods of the social sciences where these are taught in a physical sciences-health related framework. As is true with many social scientists teaching in medical faculties there is some temptation to accept the role of the 'soft' scientist who offers less 'real' data and analysis. However, the drive behind this chapter is to offer a caution to social scientists tempted to take a less assertive role in relation to physical sciences health research.

I intend to show that in the context of physical science health related research (and more specifically, research in local council health survey-ing courses) that the social sciences qualitative and quantitative research methodologies offer a fresh and innovative insight into physical sciences approaches and extend the implications of such traditional physical health research beyond its present bounds.

I will discuss two issues. First, even though a major proportion of health related research teaching has traditionally been conducted from within the physical sciences disciplines it frequently results in students who develop a fairly narrow, positivist perspective on health sciences issues. That research is limited in scope, their view of social, cultural and political implications is limited, and their understanding of the implications of the results of research is frequently narrow. In particular, students studying a health surveyor's curriculum have traditionally been disadvantaged by the limitations of the more positivist physical sciences approach to research. Second, I will illustrate how both qualitative and quantitative social sciences research methodologies can enhance the understanding that physical science trained students have. Examples of students' research will be drawn from a final year's research methods subject in a health surveyor's degree course at an Australian University of Technology.

During the past three years I have worked on developing the course in conjunction with other staff from the applied science faculty. Students who complete the course are frequently engaged by local councils in a health inspectorate role. This role has a research component and normally involves contributing to local council health policy (particularly food practices and the environment). Over the past few years the development of degree courses for health surveyors has seen the role of the local council food inspector develop into a more professional role of health surveyor. This change has seen them moving increasingly into local council policy formulation. As their professional role expands a greater demand is placed on these people to conduct research.

The course was reconstructed from a three to a four year degree programme with the inclusion of a two semester research methods and thesis component. Students are required to complete a one semester research methods subject in preparation for completing their thesis. Research projects are normally undertaken by teams of two students: in conjunction they present a thesis at the end of the second semester. Unlike many social science colleagues working in physical sciences programmes I was fortunate in that my applied sciences colleagues actively encouraged some social sciences integration into their programme.

SOCIAL SCIENCE AND PHYSICAL SCIENCE METHODOLOGY

Health issues such as the extent of water and environmental pollution, the effectiveness of medical waste disposal systems, and strategies for the eradication of mosquito populations have in the past tended to be traditionally researched from the separate perspectives of a physical sciences discipline. A traditional physical sciences approach to water pollution testing, for example, would be to selectively test water samples to determine any settings and/or times where pollution levels are over specified limits.

Other disciplines may test the social impact of polluted waterways by showing how recreational and related behaviours are influenced by not being able to use local streams or reservoirs. Rarely however is an integrated research design conducted where raw pollution figures are interpreted in their social, cultural and political context. For the health surveyor, a vital policy question might be 'what are the various implications of polluted waterways on recreational use?' However, an even more important question might be 'what impact could polluted recreational facilities have on the definition of recreation, health behaviour and the concept of a community facility for a resident group?'

A social science interview-based programme could supply information or 'fact' gathering in the health physical sciences on this kind of project. For the health surveying policy maker then, the raw facts would have a broader meaning in their social context. In such a case social science research strategy adds a substantial dimension to raw physical science topics. Physical health sciences data may have a particular meaning and implication in one context, and entirely different implications in another. Also, social sciences research methods encourage a much greater exploration of why and how 'facts' are the way that they are.

To continue with the pollution example, a creek with a pollution level above that specified as safe by the Environmental Protection Authority will have a very different consequence if there is a user population that identifies it as an important recreational facility. If the people in the area define fishing, bathing and associated activities as important to them, having the creek nearby, then the policy and strategic implications of a polluted creek are far reaching. Local residents may have purchased properties specifically for the recreational facilities provided by a creek in the area. The local councils would be required to service the creek as a resource and facility: it would be included as part of the recreational profile of the council. Council planning and policy would need to incorporate issues based on the pollution of recreational facilities.

ISSUES OF PROTOCOL

Physical sciences enquiry in the health sciences, particularly in health surveying largely involves gathering and testing data to be presented outside the context of its social meaning. The role of social science strategy is to rescue that and to recombine these with the 'facts' in which various authorities are interested. These reconstituting processes allow all interested parties to read aspects of the research within a context that gives greater cultural meaning to the findings.

While the integrative approach is in its infancy, the aim is to fully extend a social science evaluation into physical science-based projects. There have, however, already been a number of research projects conducted by students which have gone well beyond the domain of traditional physical sciences research in providing a broader social, cultural and political context within which those scientific 'facts' are gathered. This practice of giving an interpretation or broader meaning to data is seen by those students as a unique contribution of social sciences methods.

There has been a broad range of investigations using more social research approaches by students on the course. I will outline some of these in order to show the diversity of methodological approaches that have been used to extend physical sciences investigations.

Example one

In one project, students tested swimming pools for total alkalinity and pH, and total bacterial counts among other organisms. They found that only two of the 14 tested pools passed water purification standards. The students interviewed pool managers and found that their preoccupation with cleaning and other duties in their hotels helped to explain their lack of knowledge of pool disinfectant maintenance. In addition they discovered that 24-hour access by bathers meant that an adequate disinfectant checking system had not been established. Their study enabled them to discover some structural and organizational causes for inadequate levels of maintenance which led to useful conclusions about restructuring maintenance programmes.

If the study had not used social science methods it may have relied on comparisons between water purification levels gained for the different swimming pools and may have focused on questions of the adequacy of chemical treatments. The additional interview programme undertaken by students enabled them to identify a range of likely causes including role conflict and inadequate training of personnel for water purification procedures.

Example two

Another student project investigated the safety of a needle and syringe disposal programme. Normally, from an applied sciences health research position the project would have been based on an evaluation of contamination levels and the properties of needle disposal containers. The use of a social science research method did not add to the physical sciences investigation: rather it re-oriented students towards another form of investigation. In doing this it refocused their perspective for the study. They investigated the types of containers and collection systems used by local councils. Their interview with local councils broadened the physical sciences investigation to include organizational aspects of the needle disposal programme. They found through interview that the number of safely disposed needles depended on the number of containers and their location. However they found no correlation between numbers of needles and syringes disposed and council strategies to make users in communities aware of the services provided. This particular investigation would normally not have been considered by science-based students and demonstrates the flexibility of topic for investigation by using social science research techniques.

Example three

One qualitative study undertook to measure the control of the spread of communicable diseases in childcare centres. This was based on a review of research which showed growing inadequacies in the control of communicable disease transmission. The study was under-taken to examine the extent of health hazard exposure. The students undertaking the research discovered through interviewing that pathogens had been identified and enteric disease had led to outbreaks at the childcare centre studied. Rotavirus was found to be a common infection as well as conjunctivitis, smallpox, pediculoses and other minor disorders. They found that the less experienced childcare workers needed improved prevention methods.

A lack of staffing resources was found to lead to insufficient surveillance of children. They also found that ongoing education in disease detection and prevention for staff and co-ordinators was inadequate. In addition, information on communicable disease was inadequate for childcare centres. This study extended a normal physical sciences investigation which would have normally focused on the degree to which health standards were met. The social science methods provided a greater explanation of the causes of inadequate health care and prevention by explaining 'background' social factors. A number of other research projects have used qualitative and quantitative social science research strategies in investigations in the context of physical sciences research. These include a survey of non-immunization of children and perceptions of the effects of monosodium gluta-mate (MSG).

The role of the health surveyor as physical sciences health researcher has its history located in the operative role of the health inspector. This role has increased substantially to include influence over policy-making functions for health-related issues in social sciences. The influence of four year degree course training has had an important impact in elevating the role of the health surveyor at council level. The course described here is not yet fully developed.

Further increases in integrating social science research methods with traditional physical sciences health research issues can be achieved. These will have the effect of enhancing the research findings to become a sounder basis for council policy formulation. This can be achieved by social, cultural and political considerations being accounted for in research areas that have belonged traditionally to the physical sciences. Physical sciences research into water pollution, medical waste disposal, the quality of food preparation and the eradication of mosquito breeding areas have simply entailed a report of the recorded characteristics and conditions. As I argued earlier social research methodologies can give social 'meaning' or 'context' to the 'facts'. Food preparation procedures can be studied in the context of the cultural knowledge and diversity of the proprietors and customers, and social location accounting for class and other social factors, including the political consideration of local council and State Government legislatures. This added dimension can give meaning and context to the 'hard' facts gained through laboratory testing.

To introduce physical sciences students to social science methodologies, texts and other reading, materials need to be selected carefully. Giving students the confidence to launch into a new perspective and to extend the boundaries of their previous training are important in the sort of material they are presented with in the course. In the next section I will discuss some of the considerations behind the choices of these texts and readings.

TEXTBOOKS AND READINGS

The aim in selecting reading material is to bridge a gap in the training and expectations of physical sciences students and to thereby encourage them to adopt social sciences methods and perspectives. One text which substantially frees students with a rigid physical sciences methodology and encourages them to explore a wide range of research strategies and practices is Yoland Wadsworth's (1984) book. She introduces two very useful strategies from social science methods. These are:

• participant observation and the open-ended interview, together with problem definition and community participation in data collection and data dissemination;

- participation in the research process by the subjects of research; this also extends to including the dissemination of research findings to them.

Leedy (1989) overviews fairly basic research methods and gives students some fundamental philosophical and practical research issues for consideration. The text was chosen because it adequately covers the range of quantitative and qualitative methods but is sufficiently positivist and practical to have some immediate appeal to physical sciences students. It also allows them, at least initially, to see the similarities between the physical and social methods rather than the differences.

Kidder and Judd (1986) and Monette *et al.* (1990) give far more detail on sampling techniques and research design for quantitative analysis. These books were chosen as they present an eminently 'rigorous' approach to research design which appeals immediately to physical sciences students with positivist expectations about what constitutes 'real' research. They discuss experimental and quasi-experimental research designs and detailed sampling techniques which make students feel less concerned with issues of reliability, validity and general method. They help to bridge a gap in students' expectations between their trained orientation to research and the social sciences. Students, however, are also introduced to Miles and Huberman (1984) at a later stage during the course. This is an excellent text on qualitative research design and techniques and has proved particularly useful for the design of open-ended interview schedules: it shows important methods for gaining maximum value through open-ended techniques. The Miles and Huberman text acts somewhat as a point of departure for students from the rigorous 'scientific' boundaries of the physical science methods into more uncharted waters. Not all students embrace qualitative open-ended methods, but those who do often see it as a completely new area to explore, and do so with genuine enthusiasm.

Other reading for the course has been chosen because it demonstrates the rigour and sophistication of social sciences methods. De Vaus (1985) is a thorough easy-to-interpret guide to the construction of survey research and can give students confidence in the strength of methods used. One book that shows a very clear way of presenting results from quantitative analysis is Graetz and MacAllister (1988). It also introduces students to the conceptual and practical rigours of using path modelling techniques in social research. Again this is a text that most physical sciences students with a mathematics background would feel quickly at ease with. It is primarily a report of research (including numerous tables) but it also includes a description of the method employed through the text: students can easily understand why research procedures are being used. Physical sciences students can very easily learn a great deal about sophisticated social sciences quantitative techniques from this book: this can encourage them to look more quickly outside their learned method for ways of investigating.

Finally Norusis (1987), in one of her many publications shows the meaning and use of most of the statistics and other measures involving computer applications in social sciences research. This book introduces students to adapting and utilizing their own mathematics and statistics training for social sciences issues, and again reduces perceived barriers between the methods. Readers considering texts for integrating physical and social sciences research methodologies should consider the role that some books can have in leading physical sciences students to feel comfortable initially with the tools of social sciences research. Some students can make abrupt transitions, but mostly students need to develop confidence with the methods as well as the perspectives of the social sciences.

CONCLUSION

Do the implications of the integrated course described here apply only to the Australian University of Technology where it is taught, or do they apply more widely, to other types of courses in other universities and colleges? I have argued that where health sciences are taught either within medical faculties, applied science faculties or in related discipline areas, the traditional physical sciences approach can have its narrow perspective modified and its boundaries of research teaching considerably extended by social sciences. Readers who teach social sciences within those types of curricula may find that physical sciences colleagues seek justification for the methods of social science research. This can be rather annoying as it is often based on a lack of knowledge of those methods. However they can and should publicize their successes and innovations to their physical sciences colleagues in order to break down those boundaries. I would encourage them to pursue the argument that social sciences not only complement the far more limited perspectives of the physical sciences in health research, but they have an extremely important role in making their investigations thorough, rigorous and more relevant politically and ethically. That message can be driven home to physical sciences faculties only by frequent and regular demonstrations of this fact in seminars, publications and simple conversation.

If physical sciences colleagues are given greater exposure to the benefits and merits of social science contributions they are likely to lose some of their narrow preconceptions and be prepared to engage in greater dialogue about the benefits of integrated curricula. Physical sciences colleagues need to be invited to social sciences seminars to increase their exposure to the benefits of these methods: real benefits could be gained by presenting to them the unique ethical, philosophical and methodological contributions of social sciences. It also helps to work closely together on curriculum development: this gives significant opportunities to discuss preconceptions (and prejudices) that sometimes prevent physical scientists engaging in debates.

Obviously physical sciences health research provides some very important data. Its major drawcard is that it has demonstrated rigorous experimental techniques: the validity of measures is high, and reliability of research measures and results is also high. Many physical scientists however perceive the validity and reliability of social sciences methods as low. However, despite rigorous methods the relevance of much physical sciences research data can be lost without considering it in the broader context of its social meaning, cultural significance and the political implications of its findings. Social sciences methods provide a far broader spectrum of research methods for investigating problems, which can make the results of research highly relevant: its social, cultural, economic and political significance is high. The social relevance that social science perspectives provide for physical sciences research aptly and significantly increases the reliability of research findings and as such makes the social science contribution a highly valued and complementary one. It is these contributions that those of us involved in combined curricula should push home demonstrably to our physical sciences colleagues.

REFERENCES

De Vaus, D. (1985) *Surveys in Social Research*, Allen and Unwin, Sydney.

Graetz, B., and MacAllister, I. (1988) *Dimensions of Australian Society*, The MacMillan Publishing Company of Australia, Australia.

Kidder, L.H. and Judd, C.M. (1986) *Research Methods in Social Relations*, Holt, Reinhart and Winston, Inc, New York.

Leedy, P.D. (1989) *Practical Research: Planning and Design*, 4th edn, MacMillan Publishing Company, New York.

Miles, M.B. and Huberman, M. (1984) *Qualitative Data Analysis. A Source Book of New Methods*, Sage Publications, Beverly Hills.

Monette, D.R., Thomas, J.S. and Cornell, R.D. (1990) *Applied Social Science Research*, Holt, Reinhart and Winston, Inc, New York.

Norusis, M. (1987) *The SPSS Guide to Data Analysis for SPSSX*, SPSS Inc, Chicago.
Wadsworth, Y. (1984) *Do it Yourself Social Research*, Council of Social Service, Melbourne Family Care Organization, Victoria.

CHAPTER 5

The politics of method in public health research

Ian Robottom and Derek Colquhoun

INTRODUCTION

As we write this chapter we are reflecting on our experiences from an Australian health promotion conference which we recently attended in Adelaide. At that conference one of the issues that emerged was the dominance of biomedical perspectives in public health, community health, health promotion and health education. This was evidenced by the presentation of data from large-scale health promotion campaigns, the heavy use of and reliance on statistics and quantitative procedures, the dominance of language stressing 'skills', 'aims and objectives', 'targets' and 'competencies', and finally, a real pressure felt by most of the participants that validity and reliability are **the** two crucial components in any worthwhile research and that the 'real world' to strive for in developing health interventions is 'wide applicability'. Needless to say we came away from that conference a little bemused and confounded. It appeared to us that a few people at the conference shared some of these concerns (not, may we add, the male professors who tended to dominate proceedings) and that there is a real need for alternative approaches within the health research area. Of particular concern to us was the total lack of appreciation of the richness and potential of methodology – this was subsumed by a belief that the major problem with method was to improve the validity, reliability and generalizability of the 'interventions'. In this we would agree with Gitlin, Siegel and Boru (1989) who have suggested that the emphasis on reliability and validity has 'obscured the relation between method and what the research is trying to achieve through the method – its political moment'. This politics of diversion, away from the view that methodology is inherently political, has limited the extent to which the health area has adopted innovative and creative research designs. In this chapter we would like to demonstrate the point by sharing our experiences of an action research project with a group of adolescents in the environmental health area. We will begin by setting out the background and context of the project, and in subsequent sections we will discuss the assumptions underpinning the adopted methodology, and provide a contextualized account of the methodology-in-action.

BACKGROUND AND CONTEXT OF THE PROJECT

In 1989 we were visited by Bill Linford and Anne Fairbairn (two youth workers in local municipal councils). Bill and Anne approached us with the idea of an action research project to investigate health and environmental issues of concern to local young people. Bill and Anne thought that since Deakin University was a relatively large institution, money would be available to fund such research. Unfortunately that was not the case and we had to look outside the institution for funding. Several coinciding events led to our eventual success in this search.

About this time an invitation-only conference was being organized by Evan Willis and Jeanne Daly from neighbouring La Trobe University with funding from the Public Health and Medical Research Council (PHRDC) for health social scientists to share their experiences of applying for research grants. Rumour was rife amongst researchers in the area that predominantly biomedical research was being funded and the PHRDC was concerned that 'qualitative' and types of research other than biomedical should also be funded and supported. Delegates at the conference were from a variety of disciplines including sociology, anthropology and education. One outcome of the conference was the establishment of the Directory of Health Social Sciences for all those researching in the health area. A less tangible outcome was the feeling that mainly biomedical research was indeed being funded and there was also a need for possibly more creative and innovative research designs. Fortunately, a spur for us at the conference was the presentation by Yoland Wadsworth (1990) on action research.

A second incident was that Deakin University's Faculty of Education has a history of action research (Kemmis and McTaggart, 1988) so it was understandable for us to be sympathetic to what Wadsworth was advocating. Finally, the third coincidence which brought the research project to fruition was the tendering of public health research grants by the PHRDC. We brought together our cumulative experiences and decided to apply for an action research grant in the area of environmental health. We nominated our assessors who we thought would be sympathetic and eight months later the grant was awarded. Two years after the conference the PHRDC has still not funded another project similar to this one even though several proposals have been submitted. The eventual title of the project reflected our interests: 'Action Research and Adolescents' Perceptions of Environment and Health'. The project could now begin in earnest.

The adolescents involved in the project were part of the Bellarine Youth Network (BYN), a group which had formed two years previously. The BYN was established in early 1989 following a conference/camp for young people organized by Bill Linford at the Institute of Educational Administration, an independent organization close to Deakin University. The camp consisted of various activities dealing with communication and leadership skills. The idea of forming a youth network was discussed and the young people at the conference were invited to join. The original members of the BYN were from three secondary schools on the Bellarine Peninsula: Queenscliff, Newcomb and Geelong East Technical Schools. In the past three years, membership of the BYN has always been between nine and 12, although only a few of the original members remain.

In the next section we will explain some of the assumptions we feel are inherent within action research and how those assumptions have guided and influenced the project to date. In particular, we will illustrate the political nature of the research act and argue that the question of technique or method should go beyond a mere 'tools of the trade' mentality.

THE POLITICS OF METHOD: ASSUMPTIONS UNDERPINNING THE METHODOLOGY

Aside from the politics of status, control and power located in our forms of professional socialization, our social work structures, and our reward systems, the ultimate politics of method is its impact on our view of reality ... There is no such thing as a value-neutral approach to the world; language itself, whether the language of the arts or the sciences is value-laden. To acquire a language or a set of methodological conventions without examining what they leave out as well as what they can contain, is to take the part for the whole. Hence, when I talk about the politics of method, I do not simply mean matters of position, authority or professionalization in the narrow sense, but rather the ways in which the mind is shaped and beliefs are fostered. The politics of method ultimately has to do with the politics of experience. Method influences how we think and what we are permitted to feel. (Eisner, 1988.)

It should come as no surprise then, that we view research methodology as inherently problematic. We take our ideas predominantly from critical social science and in particular the work of Carr and Kemmis (1986) who have applied several fundamental assumptions of critical social science to education research. In this section we will outline these assumptions and later we will consider the way they have been worked through in practice in our project.

Elsewhere (Robottom and Colquhoun, 1992) we have characterized the rationale for our choice of methodology as three distinct approaches to research in the social sciences: research **on** other people (traditional 'positivistic' research); research **for** other people ('interpretive and enlightening' research); and the approach we prefer, collaborative research **with other social actors** (action research). This simple trichotomy of research approaches is simplistic but it does serve to highlight the many assumptions and key issues underpinning the selection of research methodology. According to Carr and Kemmis (1986) there are five assumptions underpinning research in the critical social sciences, and any adequate approach:

- must reject positivist notions of rationality, objectivity and truth;
- must accept the need to employ the interpretive categories of the social actors involved;
- must provide ways of distinguishing ideologically distorted interpretations from those that are not. It must also provide some view of how any distorted self-understanding is to be overcome;
- must be concerned to identify and expose those aspects of the existing social order which frustrate the pursuit of rational goals and must be able to offer theoretical accounts which make social actors aware or how they may be eliminated or overcome;
- must be pratical.

Critical social science research in this 'postpositivist world' (Anderson, 1989) problematizes views which see technical and instrumental solutions to social issues. In particular, objectivity and value neutrality are questioned and laid bare. We also need to adopt a perspective which allow us to elicit the meanings of the social actors with whom we are working. In this way the research is grounded in the real life experiences of the participants rather than by an outside 'expert' detailing significant moments in the research process. In addition, we must use these grounded experiences and meanings to interrogate and distinguish ideologically distorted perceptions of reality. According to Carr and Kemmis (1986) this may be akin to what Freire has termed 'conscientization' (Freire, 1970). Indeed, in our project these assumptions were conceived as:

being concerned with (i) helping social actors in the identification of various perceptions and meanings of life so that vested interests in the definition of environment and health can be conceptualized as **problematic**, (ii) helping to raise **consciousness** about the environmental and health values already existing in public health strategies; and then (iii) helping social actors to **act** more appropriately in the light of their environmental and health values (Robottom and Colquhoun, 1992).

Action research too should be conceptualized as problematic. If we failed to reflect on our experiences and practices then we would not be true to the spirit of the action research process. With this in mind and to aid in our reflections, we have borrowed another set of assumptions, this time from Max van Manen (1990).

Van Manen asserts that the basic assumptions underpinning action research are usually taken for granted and rarely questioned, and our belief in them may led to 'false victories, strange contradictions and confounding failures'. These assumptions include:

- the democracy assumption;
- the external knowledge assumption;
- the reflection/action assumption;
- the change assumption;
- the teacher (or participant) as researcher assumption.

At the heart of all action research projects is the belief that power (however it is manifest) should be shared equally among participants. There is no sense of the researcher researching 'subjects'. The use of democratic language reinforces this point and subjects become participants who are actively involved in decision making from the start of the project and at every step in the process. Allied to this is the role of the visiting expert who may approach research in a 'rape and pillage' fashion: taking what he or she wants for his or her own purposes and leaving behind a trail of mayhem and destruction. The expert's role in action research is often one that shifts through several phases from that of 'technical' support, such as providing advice on data gathering techniques, through to a more educational role involving acting as facilitators and moderators and eventually as co-researchers and participants. As Kemmis (1990) has noted:

- We began to understand more clearly what it means to say that in the process of critical action research, there is room only for participants. In genuinely critical and self-critical research, all participants must take on genuinely collaborative roles, as members of, not outsiders to, the research work, even if roles within the group are differentiated. The projects should be collaborative projects governed by open discussion making in a group committed to examining its own values, understandings, practices, forms of organization and situation.

Another cornerstone of action research is that it involves a change in the social conditions in which social actors find themselves, and a change in the activities of those particular social actors. Action research projects in education for example are often involved with the improvement of professional practice (teaching) and the improvement of the conditions in which that practice occurs. Clearly, there is a whole range of changes that could be made through reflecting and acting, for example, at the 'technical' end of the continuum we may see an improvement in how a teacher assesses students but at the 'broader' socio-cultural end of the continuum we may see an improvement in the teacher's ability to change the dominant rationale and context for assessment and perhaps the way in which assessment is often used as a form of social control. Of course, inherent within action research is the mandate that participants themselves must be involved in the research process of planning, reflection and action. It is impossible to 'do' action research 'to' other people (although we are sure some may have tried). Participants need to be central to any action research project so that their meanings, perceptions and experiences are fundamental to the process.

In the next section of this chapter we will indicate how these assumptions from both Kemmis and van Manen have influenced our National Health and Medical Research Council (NH and MRC) action research project into adolescents' perceptions of environment and health. Also, by working through these related assumptions we will illustrate (not necessarily using the terminology of Kemmis and van Manen) other issues such as co-optability of the research, identity, ownership, control and empowerment.

THE POLITICS OF METHOD: THE ENACTMENT OF THE METHODOLOGY

The Bellarine Youth Network (BYN) formed out of a perceived need for young people to have some kind of representation in decision-making processes, particularly those decisions concerning young people made by the local council. It was felt that there was a lack of understanding of the needs of young people by the decision makers and the provision of services to meet those needs. Individuals have joined the BYN for a variety of reasons but a common reason has been the desire to achieve something positive for young people. At the very least the BYN raises issues concerning young people and tries to communicate their needs and concerns to the decision makers in the local community. Prior to the commencement of the action research project the BYN has been involved in many activities, discussed many issues and has become well known in the region for being involved with other groups and agencies. Of particular note and relevance to this project are the BYN's activities concerning the issue of sewage disposal along the local surf coast. The BYN consulted local groups with interests in the quality of the coastal environment such as the 'Sewage Surfriders' and the 'Australian Environmental Security Force' and had access to information collected by Queenscliff High School on the *E. coli* levels at local beaches. The BYN invited the public, representatives from the Department of Fisheries and Wildlife and the Geelong and District Water Board and various pressure groups to an open forum to discuss the sewage treatment plant responsible for the pollution. Other issues addressed by the BYN have included the lack of transport facilities on the Peninsula, under age drinking and the lack of entertainment for young people.

Without pre-empting the discussion to follow it is possible to outline several of the key issues or substantive concerns which have merged so far throughout the present action research project. These concerns have arisen through the interactions of the BYN at meetings and at other forums such as presentations to interested agencies and groups such as community health workers. In all, five strongly related issues have been identified by the members of the project as worthy of initial research including stress from schoolwork, the role of young people in community action, the problems of ownership of and commitment to the project, the role of advertising, and the role of groups such as the BYN in communicating with other youth groups. These issues are presented here but they are in their formative stages and we recognize that the issues will change both in substance and form throughout the project.

The issue of greatest concern to the BYN appears to be that of stress induced by schoolwork. In particular the stress brought about by the introduction of the new state-based Victorian Certificate in Education (VCE). The VCE was recently introduced by the Ministry of Education in Victoria following a Ministerial statement from the then Minister of Education, the Hon. Ian Cathie. According to Kirner (1989) this statement, *Future Directions in Post Compulsory Schooling*, outlined the plans for the introduction of the VCE and highlighted concerns with the pre-VCE education system. These concerns included the proliferation of units available to students, the lack of choice of subjects, the different assessment methods for different subjects, the problems of comparability of results and the inadequate preparation of the students for work and further study. The VCE was conceptualized as the solution to these problems in *The Blackburn Report*, which concentrated on the post-compulsory years of schooling (Kirner, 1989).

Unfortunately the switch from the old High School Certificate (HSC) to the new VCE has not been unproblematic. The young people in the project were consistently concerned with the **quantity** of work involved in the VCE and not necessarily with the **quality** of work needed to be submitted. The VCE involves two years of continual assessment instead of the old HSC 'do-or-die' examination. Assessment is usually a combination of externally marked examinations together with individual student projects. Students are now faced with deadlines throughout the two years of grades 11 and 12 (the equivalent of age 17 and 18 or A levels in England, Wales and Northern Ireland). This constant pressure to perform is the source of much of the stress felt by the young members of the BYN. The significant aspect of stress of course is that it does not just affect the adolescents' schoolwork – it filters right through to all spheres of their lives including their family life, relationships with members of the opposite sex, work after school and their recreation time. Of particular concern to members of the BYN has been the way in which stress has been individualized by the schools on the Peninsula. Stress has been conceptualized very much as a matter of time management – manage your time, keep to deadlines, prepare well in advance and be methodical and systematic, learn to study correctly and efficiently and you will not be stressed. Unfortunately all this approach appears to do is compound the problem. Members of the BYN do not want their stress to be exacerbated by being blamed for not having the 'correct' study skills or time management skills. At the time of writing the BYN are considering what options are open to them in terms of responding to the problem of VCE stress. There are plans for a statewide conference run by the BYN for young people on the issue of stress at school.

Allied to this of course is the extent of the active role that young people can play in community action projects. Clearly, if young people are busy with schoolwork or too 'stressed out' from this schoolwork then it will be difficult if not impossible for these young people living on the Peninsula to become actively engaged in community action. Some of the concerns expressed by members of the project include issues of advocacy and empowerment (to which we will return later) and the role of their schoolwork in delimiting the extent of this social action. Is schoolwork for instance, simply another form of social control bearing in mind the huge percentages of young people now staying on at school to grades 11 and 12?

Early in the life of the action research project, the adult participants were keen to emphasize that the BYN members 'owned' the project. Clearly, the university 'chief investigators' have a responsibility to the university and the NH and MRC, if only for forecasting the budget. However, there was much more at stake than the mere technicalities of spending the research money. In particular, there were concerns about the relationships between the adult members of the BYN and the adolescent members. As Lynne Stevens, the PhD student working on the project, has commented in her discussion notes:

> At first the Deakin personnel were at pains to stand back and 'let it happen' (some more so than others) which resulted in frustration for all involved because not much did happen. This emphasis on ownership seemed to cause uncertainty because the BYN members were not sure how to proceed in what was new territory for them and they seemed to be looking for guidance from the adult members of the project. Bill Linford's changed role (from instigator to facilitator) seemed to cause uncertainty as to how to proceed as he always took an active part in proceedings. This points to the fragile nature of 'participatory research' with a group that is relatively powerless.

The original submission to the NH and MRC involved a critique of the role of the media in forming the attitudes of young people to environmental health issues. The role of advertising was another focus for discussion by the members of the BYN, in particular those advertisements that encouraged risk reducing behaviours such as stopping smoking, drinking less (and with more control), and saying no to drugs. These advertisements were often part of national campaigns but their efficacy was cast in doubt after one meeting of the BYN where members professed to be immune from advertising and they suggested that their behaviour was in no way influenced by the media. This left all of us unsure about the role of the media in health promotion and especially in the areas of attitude formation or change. It was suggested at one meeting that the reporting of VCE stress in the media might be a source of research for the group.

The final issue of concern to the BYN was that covering communication with other groups in the community. The question which was posed at one meeting was concerned with the role of a group such as the BYN in informing, directing and changing the discussions among young people and other constituencies in the communities about environmental health issues of concern and interest to them. Some other questions raised included: Do the communication channels established by community groups have any lasting existence or are they one-offs (are they sustainable)? Are the communication channels independent of the substantive issues (in the case of environmental health) that they were originally set up to serve? Is there any evidence of these channels of communication being effective in improving discourse about important issues?

The idea of 'participation' was foremost in our minds in the early days of the project. It was thought to be important for the adolescent members of the BYN to actually be involved in doing research. We thought we understood that it was imperative for the focus of such research to be environmental or health issues of interest or concern to the BYN members themselves, as opposed, say, to issues that we as adults had a specific interest in. So one of the first things we did was to invite an acknowledged overseas expert in interviewing techniques to come along and speak about this research technique to the BYN meeting. The expert, from the Centre for Applied Research in Education at the University of East Anglia in England, gave an account of the rationale, techniques, and contextualized examples of interviewing as an instrument in ethnographic research. On the basis of the ideas on interviewing that came out of this meeting, we agreed that members of the BYN should begin an interview-based survey of the environmental and health perceptions of their peers in a range of school and recreational contexts. To our dismay, the outcome of this was something of a disaster.

The adolescent members of the BYN reported feeling uncomfortable about the formal interviewing of their peers, and they perceived similar feelings of discomfort among the interviewees. They reported a reluctance among interviewees to address seriously the task of articulating environmental and health issues. It was decided to discontinue this activity as there was a general feeling that we were 'spinning our heels' (i.e. we were spending a lot of time talking about a form of data collection that simply was not working).

Our own diary notes on this episode show our reaction to the experience:

> It is clear that we may not have been sensitive to the 'real' issues affecting this group. We have become aware that the discourse at BYN meetings might have been driven more by our methodological agenda (of wanting interviews to occur for the sake of the research, etc.) than by a substantive agenda of issues of real interest and concern to the young people. That is, we had become aware of a need to 'internalize the research agenda'. After the last meeting of 13 August, perhaps we see that our own vested interest in wishing to pursue recognizable (to us) health or environmental issues of a more traditional kind (like Black Rock, or availability of STD clinics) has clouded our perceptions of perhaps the most pressing issue for these people – that of VCE-related stress. We now need to see this issue as an environmental health issue (it implicates the 'environment' of the VCE/schooling context; and it definitely has health considerations for those experiencing stress within this context).
>
> As such this issue is a proper and legitimate topic for discussion and action within BYN meetings in particular and the NH

and MRC project in general. It is a topic that we probably should explore through reports of personal experience from the BYN members and investigation of support strategies within schools and the community.

The research question now may be: 'How can the research act as a supportive enterprise for these kids in the VCE predicament? How can we ensure that discussion of the VCE-stress issue is seen as legitimate in project meetings?' (Research Meeting).

In a sense, we see our early interest in peer interviewing as a 'preoccupation with method' that may be quite widespread in efforts in participatory research. A preoccupation with method in this case expressed itself as a commitment to interviewing on the grounds that to do interviewing was to be seen to be doing research. In particular, the reliability and validity of interviewing (even though we did not use those terms) were of prime concern to the BYN members, who wanted to be certain that they were all asking the 'right questions' in the 'right way'. This concentration of our efforts on issues of reliability and validity, in retrospect, led to a 'politics of diversion', where substantive issues concerning environment and health, plus, more importantly, political issues concerning the methodology were marginalized and/or neglected. Kemmis and DiChiro (1987), in describing action research projects conducted at Deakin University in Australia and elsewhere, aptly expressed the kind of situation we found ourselves in.

> Those involved at the core of a project have found themselves acting in ways which treat others as objects of their action – for example, trying to 'get' others to 'feel ownership' of problems (rather than starting from the concerns and problems which they already 'own', or to put it less proprietorially, starting from their concerns) or trying to 'get' others involved in the process. This way of thinking about action research reveals a preoccupation with problems of 'method' or 'technique': action research, on this view, has been de-problematized and reified. The action research method becomes a routine which others are to follow.

It turned out that our 'preoccupation with method' had, in a sense, blinded us to some issues that were emerging more authentically, independently of our well-intentioned attempts to 'make research happen'. As we commented earlier some of these issues have been documented elsewhere (Robottom and Colquhoun, 1992), and are summarized here.

Establishing identity

Participants in this project are committed to establishing their own group identity. The members of the BYN initiated the idea of BYN lapel badges and identity cards. The members of the BYN have been strong in their advocacy of rotating chairpersonship and shared secretarial duties; members of the BYN saw the fact that they did not have a permanent chairperson (especially an adult) as a feature distinguishing their group from similar youth groups elsewhere in the region. They retained control over the process of gaining publicity for the project – they contributed to the development of a press release, were interviewed by reporters from the local press, and organized a live interview on community radio. The word association activity was their means of establishing their own conception of 'environment' and 'health' – a means of clarifying their own beginning positions on these topics. However, it should be noted that this interest in identity does not reflect a singular notion of what that identity should be – as could be expected in a social group of this kind, there are emerging differences and even contests about the nature of identity and purpose.

The politics of relationships and the problem of ownership

Adolescent members of the BYN are receiving money out of the research grant allocation. The BYN members themselves are the gatekeepers to the annual installments that the NH and MRC (via the university personnel) make to the project each year from the original grant. These annual installments can be disbursed in ways deemed to be appropriate by members of the BYN. A BYN member is treasurer, and another is signatory to the account. An issue remains about whether payment, however it is mediated, improves the 'professional' status of participants' research or simply rewards instrumental contributions to our own research agenda. That is, are the members of the BYN simply research assistants for the university personnel? The act itself of paying the members of the BYN does nothing to redress any power relationship that exists between university personnel and BYN members; making these payments may actually reinforce the power relationships, since only the co-ordinators (the university personnel) are in a position to choose to act in this way. Similarly, the research attempts consciously to withdraw from imposing an 'expert' or other peer power relationship – but this again may serve to actually reinforce the power relationship, since only the university personnel have the power to make this decision. A continuing methodological issue that we need to recognize and work through is the tension between the valuing of participatory research on the one hand and the idea of 'university expertise' on the other.

Another danger is that efforts to maintain a critical methodological self-consciousness might slide into indeterminate self-indulgence.

Co-optability of participatory research

We know from involvement in other participatory research projects that there may come a time in participatory research when participants exercise the principle of an 'internal research agenda' by strongly asserting their control over the direction of the research. There may be attempts by participants to co-opt the research to serve their own interests as they perceive them within the flux of changing power relationships of which they form an active part. From the vantage point of conventional applied-science (experimental) approaches to research, this may be seen as undesirable – co-optation of the research by participants can, on this view, be denigrated. But if participatory research is to enact distinctive ideology, it seems that this co-option of the research by participants is a **necessary** moment. The moment when participants recognize the research itself as an instrument of empowerment should be celebrated rather than denigrated. On the other hand, a methodological dilemma would arise if the redirection of the research was seen as simply reinforcing a different set of power relationships that are just as oppressive as the ones they replace (the issue of who could ever be in a position to make these kinds of judgements remains problematic).

THE FOREST AND THE TREES: ACKNOWLEDGING PARTICIPATORY RESEARCH

A year into the project, we want to acknowledge an irony: we suggest that our preoccupation with method has prevented us from seeing that participatory research has been going on all along. If we were to set out the process of this research, it would be in the following terms (acknowledging that the process is more interactive than the somewhat linear description implied by standard paragraph construction).

- The adolescent members of the BYN encounter in their everyday school and recreational activities and interactions a number of perspectives held by their peers in respect of environment and health. These perspectives are 'picked up' incidentally rather than as a result of any organized interview survey strategy.
- At fortnightly BYN meetings, usually of three hours' duration, all participants are asked to make a verbal report of the kinds of environmental and health perspectives and issues that they have

encountered in the period between meetings. In addition, participants from time to time bring examples of press articles that are analysed for their implicit or explicit perspectives on environment and health. The research assistant also collects and brings to meetings news cuttings about environmental and health issues on the Bellarine Peninsula. There is great variation in the way in which these processes of reporting and analysis take place – it is certainly an informal process, often taking place at the same time as enormous quantities of pizza and soft drinks are consumed.

- These informal reports of young people's perceptions of environmental and health issues in their community and outcomes of analysis of news cuttings are recorded in minutes of the meetings. In addition, the project's research assistant interviews participants on a regular basis and transcripts of these interviews add to the developing 'database'.
- The university-based researchers develop sets of 'working notes' from this database of meeting reports and interview transcripts, in which the fairly disparate collection of recorded perspectives are anonymized and organized loosely around particular issues. These working notes are distributed to participants, who appraise them in terms of their fairness, relevance and accuracy.
- The working notes are ultimately further developed by the university-based researchers into a smaller number of more solid working papers, which represent a more argued account of certain issues. These working papers are again returned to participants for vetting.
- Throughout this process, the adolescent members of the BYN and the youth worker are in continual contact with other young people in the region – the adolescents through their everyday school and recreational activities, and the youth worker through his professional activities. Through the informal interactions of these activities, as well as through more formal means such as school committee structures, council meetings, and (increasingly) invitations to make presentations to various community agencies, participants make increasingly developed contributions to community discourse about current, relevant environmental and health issues.

What should we make of this kind of process? We argue that this process has a strongly educational character, for ourselves as researchers, for the adolescent members of the BYN and the youth worker as they juxtapose their own perceptions of health and environment with those of their colleagues and peers, and for the community engaged by project participants. We would also argue that the process is a form of participatory research in the terms of the assumptions set out earlier in the chapter.

In our view, a minimum achievement of participatory research is the description of a social setting. Participants in this project routinely describe (present perspectives about) local, current environmental and health issues. Of course, the descriptions presented at BYN meetings are, like any verbal description, couched in the language of the sub-culture and so are structured and interpretive in nature. As Anderson (1989) puts it, we would 'share with interpretivist ethnographers the view that the cultural informant's perceptions of social reality are themselves theoretical constructs. That is, although the informant's constructs are ... more 'experience-near' than the researcher's, they are, themselves, reconstructions of social reality'.

Like any social setting, those described by the members of the BYN are constituted of a number of power relationships, in which there are relatively more powerful groups (for example, school principals, teachers, shire councils officers, health education administrators, university personnel) and relatively less powerful groups (for example, the young people of the Bellarine Peninsula). Any description and definition of such power relationships is political, at least in the sense that description of the relationships makes them more public and hence more open to scrutiny and to changes in the distribution of power. One of the important early matters to be addressed in the project was to bring these power issues out into the open, to address and perhaps redress some of the relationships that the project had some control over at the time, for example, chairpersonship and minute taking.

The project seeks to study the 'legitimating mechanisms' in terms of which adolescents' perceptions of environment and health are intelligible. As Anderson (1990) describes it, such study requires not only close scrutiny of such traditional symbolic fare as language, myths and rituals, but also means seeking symbolic meaning in organiza-tional boundaries, structures, regulations, and policies. A critical constructivist approach acknowledges that social structures of class, patriarchy, and race exist but also asserts that they are created, sustained, and reproduced through ideologies that – if we know where to look – become visible at the symbolic level (Anderson, 1990).

The project does not treat such constructed categories as 'environ-ment' and 'health' as unproblematic, but attempts to expose their ideological aspects and the interests that are served through their reproduction or reconstruction. For example, the project is interested in problematizing environmental health by examining the ways in which the print medium acts as an agent in reproducing and reconstructing such categories of 'environment' and 'health' for public consumption. One of the questions being addressed by the project is whether the media offer a virtual reflection of 'environment' and 'health' as would a mirror, or whether our daily diet of messages about 'environment' and 'health' is more like a stew prepared by some powerful chef with a fondness for certain ingredients but not for others – that is, whether the public receives a 'constructed' stereotype.

The project will examine the way the media (especially the print medium) report developments and achievements relating to environment and health. It will collect instances of such reporting, and appraise these in terms of the particular views of environment and health that such reporting reflects, sustains or reconstructs. The development of a selection of actual news stories will be 'tracked' over time to explore the way in which the media reconstructs the issues being reported. Some of the specific research questions that the project may end up addressing are:

- In what sense does media coverage offer a virtual reflection of environment and health 'out there'?
- How does such reporting influence our images of environment and health?
- Which audiences are affected by these stories?
- In what sense are the images of environment and health available in the media reconstructed with a view to serving audiences of particular kinds? Whose versions of reality are these reconstructions serving?
- Are certain filtering principles operating in the reporting of environment and health: for example, is disease under-reported as a factor in death relative to factors of a violent and catastrophic nature?
- To what extent do environment and health journalists cover environment and health in ways that reflect their own personal interests and capabilities?
- How do environment and health journalists respond when they are in a position of needing to make a judgement between a number of competing truth claims?
- Is there a sense in which the scientists' need for public visibility is responsible for a symbiotic if not hegemonic relationship between scientists and journalists?
- What are the needs and 'rules' of professional environmental or health associations and professional journalist and media associations that influence environment and health reporting?
- What are the backgrounds and credentials of environment and health journalists?
- What standards of evidence and validity do environment and health journalists employ in their environment and health reporting?
- What proportion of media environment and health reporting is substantially error-free?
- Under what conditions does media coverage of environment and health have a pronounced impact on audiences?

- Whose interests are served by the views of environment and health being reproduced by media?

We envisage the relationship between the adolescents and the media to a be a major focus for our investigations in the remaining time of the project. The media is clearly significant in our constructions and interpretations of 'health' and 'environment' and by becoming involved in media analysis of these categories we will hopefully be able to collectively deconstruct our meanings and also be critical about our behaviour in the health and environment areas.

CONCLUSION

In this chapter we have illustrated the political nature of research in public health. By describing an action research project into adolescents' perceptions of environmental health we have demonstrated that a preoccupation with technical aspects of method(s) may simply serve to detract from the political moment in the research process. Adolescents can indeed make significant contributions to research in the environmental health area and participatory research is a real and viable alternative to the dominant and more traditional quantitative or positivistic research which subordinates adolescents to a minor instrumental role. Also, we feel we have been true to our belief that we need to report the complexities and idiosyncracies of the research process. By doing this we would support and encourage others to become involved in this type of research. We see this as an important time in the challenge to dominant perspectives in the public health area. By unearthing the complexities and idiosyncracies of the research process we feel we have given the reader a much more vivid and 'alive' interpretation of what it is to do public health research.

ACKNOWLEDGEMENT

We would like to acknowledge the valuable contributions of Lynne Stevens and Sally Lindros to the project. The project has also been financially supported by Deakin University.

REFERENCES

Anderson, G.L. (1989) Critical ethnography in education: origins, current status and new directions, *Review of Educational Research*, **59** (3), pp. 249–70.

Anderson, G. (1990) Toward a critical constructivist approach to school administration: invisibility, legitimation, and the study of non-events. *Educational Administration Quarterly*, **26** (1), pp. 38–59.

Carr, W. and Kemmis, S. (1986) *Becoming Critical: Education, Knowledge and Action Research*, Deakin University Press, Geelong.

Eisner, E. (1988) The primacy of experience and the politics of method, *Educational Research*, June/July, pp. 15–20.

Freire, P. (1970) *Cultural Action for Freedom*, Centre for the Study of Change, Cambridge, Mass.

Gitlin, A., Siegel, M. and Boru, K. (1990) The politics of method: from leftist ethnography to educative research, *Qualitative Studies in Education*, **2** (3), pp. 237–53.

Kemmis, S. (1990) *Curriculum, contestation and change: essays on education*, Deakin University Mimeograph.

Kemmis, S. and DiChiro, G. (1987) Emerging and evolving issues of action research praxis: an Australian perspective, *Peabody Journal of Education*, **64** (3), pp. 101–30.

Kemmis, S. and McTaggart, R. (eds) (1988) *The Action Research Planner*, Deakin University Press, Geelong.

Kirner, J. (1989) Ministerial statement on the VCE, *Education Victoria*, December, pp. 13–14.

Minutes of a Research Meeting held 13 August 1992.

Robottom, I. and Colquhoun, D. (1992) Participatory research, health education and the politics of method, *Health Education Research: Theory and Practice* **7** (4), pp. 457–69.

Van Manen, M. (1990) Beyond assumptions: shifting the limits of action research, *Theory into Practice*, **XXIX** (3), pp. 152–7.

Wadsworth, Y. (1990) Participant action research, *The Social Sciences and Health Research* (eds Daly, J. and Willis, E.), Public Health Association, Sydney.

CHAPTER 6

Dilemmas in cross-cultural action research

Robin McTaggart

INTRODUCTION

Studying other cultures is often regarded as an exploitative activity. All too often, Western researchers from wealthy institutions make objects of people and practices in foreign cultures in ways which more obviously serve the advancement of Western academic careers than the interests of the people studied. 'Cross-cultural action research', 'participatory (action) research' and parallel movements like 'action anthropology' were methodological efforts to try to make Western researchers' work more responsive to the concerns of people in other cultures. These participatory action research efforts addressed some of the more obvious concerns about exploitation, but raise another round of even more complex issues which are still methodological and which cannot be separated from the content of the programs in which the research activity occurs. Though participatory action research has roots in both First and Third World contexts (Kemmis and McTaggart, 1988b; Fals Borda and Rahman, 1991) the contents with which it is engaged (such as medicine, agriculture, health education, and educa- tion generally) tend to be Western in their orientation. Participatory action researchers argue that provided relationships between programme participants are openly and explicitly dialogical with commitments to symmetry and reciprocity in discourse, practice and social organization, then that is the best which can be done to offset the potential danger of Western cultural imperialism. Further, they argue that this 'best' is a superior moral alternative to staying at one's desk in the academy.

In this chapter I want to realize four general aims:

- to provide some insight into the nature of participatory action research as it is understood in the Deakin University Action Research Group;

- to draw on two examples from personal experience, one from health education in the Sudan (a project which collapsed because of cultural differences) and one from Aboriginal teacher education in Australia (a project which was 'successful' but which remains problematic in several ways), to explore some of the substantive, ethical and political issues in cross-cultural participatory action research;
- to question the aspirations of Westerners to make contact with the Third World in 'culturally sensitive' ways, and to suggest that Westerners have more to learn than they have to teach; and
- to suggest that it is Westernism itself which needs to be rethought because experience with other cultures shows that Western aid and development express an ideology which is economistic, patriarchal, individualistic, Judeo-Christian, ethnocentric and Western democratic, with moral idealism subordinated to materialism.

THE IDEA OF ACTION RESEARCH

At one level of analysis, the idea of participatory action research is straightforward enough. The first advocate of 'action research' in the English language, social psychologist Kurt Lewin (1946, 1952), described action research as proceeding in a spiral of steps, each of which is composed of planning, action, observation and the evaluation of the result of the action. However, it is a mistake to think that following the 'action research spiral' slavishly constitutes 'doing action research'. Action research is not a 'method' or a 'procedure' but a series of commitments to observe and problematize through practice the general principles described in summary here. In practice, the process begins with a general idea that some kind of improvement or change is desirable. In deciding just where to begin making improvements, a group identifies an area where members perceive a cluster of problems of mutual concern and consequence. The group decides to work together on a 'thematic concern', but to change things they must confront the culture of the institution (or programme) they work in (Kemmis and McTaggart, 1988a, McTaggart, 1991).

The cyclic nature of the Lewinian approach recognizes the need for action plans to be flexible and responsive. It recognizes that, given the complexity of real social situations, in practice it is never possible to anticipate everything that needs to be done. Lewin's deliberate overlapping of action and reflection was designed to allow changes in plans for action as the people involved learned from their own experience. Put simply, action research is the way groups of people can organize the conditions under which they can learn from their own experience, and make this experience accessible to others. That is, action research is not merely about learning, it is about knowledge production and about the improvement of practice in socially committed groups. Two of the ideas which were crucial in Lewin's work were the ideas of *group decision* and *commitment to improvement*. A distinctive feature of participatory action research is that those affected by planned changes have the primary responsibility for deciding on courses of critically informed action which seem likely to lead to improvement, and for evaluating the results of strategies tried out in practice (Kemmis and McTaggart, 1988a, McTaggart, 1991a).

In short then, we can say that action research is a form of self-reflective enquiry undertaken by participants in social situations in order to improve the rationality, justice, coherence and satisfactoriness of (a) their own social practices, (b) their understanding of these practices, and (c) the institutions and programs in which these practices are carried out. Action research has an individual aspect – action researchers change themselves, and a collective aspect – action researchers work with others to achieve change and to understand what it means to change. Action research involves participants in planning action (on the basis of reflection); in implementing these plans in their own action; in observing systematically this process; and in evaluating their actions in the light of evidence as a basis for further planning and action, and so on through a self-reflective spiral.

Action research groups are not always homogenous in composition. Most often they involve people from some work site (like a community development program) and a support institution (like a university). I will use the term **participatory** action research deliberately from here on to bring together two traditions, that of action research (in the Lewinian tradition) and that of participatory research, which has its origins in community development movements in the Third World especially (McTaggart, 1991a; 1991c). Participatory action research engages people from the academy and the workplace in an entirely different relationship. For simplicity, I will use the terms 'academic' and 'worker' to label the two groups of people typically engaged in participatory action research, though it is obvious that both terms are too narrow for the diversity of agencies and people who collaborate in participatory action research projects. I make the distinction because it helps to show the common project of participatory action researchers, as well as the distinctive roles they may play in their own institutional and cultural contexts. It is also appropriate to add a word of caution: the distinction between academics and workers must not be taken to imply a distinction between 'theoreticians' and 'practitioners' as if theory resided in one place and its implementation in another. Such a view is the antithesis of the commitment of participatory action research which seeks the development of theoretically informed practice for all parties involved.

Academics and workers in participatory action research are joined by a thematic concern – a commitment to inform and improve a particular **practice**. The use of the term 'practice' can be confusing. MacIntyre (1981) used it in the broad sense to embrace all kinds of **work** under the rubric of something like 'education'. This sense of 'practice' includes theory, organization and practice in Habermas' (1972, 1974) terms and Foucault's (1973) language, life and labour terms (discourse, organization, practice, language, relationships, activities). Obviously, the term 'practice' is sometimes used for situation-specific patterns of deliberate activity. The context will usually make it clear in which of these two general senses the term is being used, but sometimes action research lapses into, or is coopted into, instrumentalism because of this confusion. Practice sensibly conceived is not a technical activity but 'any coherent and complex form of socially established co-operative activity' (MacIntrye, 1981) with the intention 'that human powers to achieve excellence, and human conceptions of the goods and ends involved, are systematically extended' (MacIntrye, 1981). In this sense, practices like education and social work are distinguished from the institutions like schools and programs which are created to enable and protect them. This broad view of practice and the location of practices in historically formed institutions enables us to identify the common and distinct contributions participatory action researchers must make from their different institutional and cultural contexts. Academics and workers may join forces to improve the theory and practice of education, social welfare, agriculture, health, usually in the workers' own work context.

The common project of participatory action research has several aspects. Each participant, academic and worker, must undertake:

• to improve his or her own work;
• to collaborate with others engaged in the project (academics and workers) to help them improve their work; and
• to collaborate with others in their own separate (academic and worker) institutional and cultural contexts to create the possibility of more broadly informing the common project, as well as to create the material and political conditions necessary to sustain the common project and its work.

That is, participatory action research is concerned simultaneously with changing **individuals**, on the one hand, and, on the other, the **culture** of the groups, institutions and societies to which they belong. The culture of a group can be defined in terms of the characteristic substance and forms of the language and discourses, activities and practices, and social relationships and organization which constitute the interactions of the group (see Foucault, 1973; Kemmis and McTaggart, 1988a).

- The individual is a bearer of language, but 'comes to' language, as it were, finding it pre-formed as an aspect of the culture of a group or society; language 'contains' expressive and communicative potential, and the way we use language can only be changed by also changing social 'agreements' about how language is used – patterns of language use which are a first aspect of the culture of the group.
- The individual is an actor, but his or her acts are framed and understood in a social context of interaction; changing social action usually requires also changing the ways others interact with us – patterns of interaction which are a second aspect of the culture of the group.
- The individual defines himself or herself partly through his or her relationships with others, but the nature and significance of these social relationships is to be understood against the fabric of social relationships which characterize wider groups, institutions and societies; changing social relationships usually requires that others also change their perspectives on the ways we relate to them and how our relationships with them fit into the broader fabric of relationships which structure society – patterns of relationship which are a third aspect of the culture of a group.

In participatory action research, the culture of three kinds of 'group' is subject to influence: the culture of the group of academics and its extension into the academic workplace; the culture of the collaborative participatory action research group itself; and the culture of the workers' workplace and its extension into the community.

ANALYSING THE CULTURE OF WORK

Individual identity and **institutional culture** (and the forms of work made possible) come about by complex processes of **contestation**, the general form of which is expressed in Figure 6.1.

The institutionalization of particular kinds of social practice occurs through **contestation**. Some activities are chosen and reshaped ahead of others through an essentially political process. Clearly the development of social practice cannot be achieved by looking for example at 'caring', 'advocacy', or 'teaching' practice alone. Particular forms of words are selected and invented to form the discourse of the institution or programme; particular kinds of activities are selected and constructed to form the practice of the institution or programme; and particular

SOCIAL MEDIUM		INSTITUTIONAL FORM
Language	INSTITUTIONALIZATION	Discourse
Activities		Practice
	CONTESTATION	
Social relations (power)		Organization

Fig. 6.1 Registers of culture and change.

kinds of social relationship are selected and constituted to form the organization of the institution or programme. It is relatively easy to see that there can be enormous disjunctions between the social medium of ordinary community life and the organizational form of the institution or programme (especially where domination by bureaucratic edict has characterized the outcome of contestation). The resultant disjunctions may not only be destructive for the culture necessary for thoughful and informed work, but also for the individual.

The development of the work in question can be enhanced through the **identification of contradictions** which arise across and within registers within the social medium, within the institutional forms and through the dialectical process of institutionalization and contestation. Contradictions may not be immediately self-evident. It may be that the striking ordinariness and constancy of custom, habit and tradition obscure the inconsistencies which provide the stimulus to constructive action. Action researchers need look more carefully at their work than ordinary people do. The fundamental modus operandi of participatory action research is to study and analyse contradictions which arise through participants' collectively observed and self-reflectively informed efforts to improve things.

In cross-cultural contexts, the identification of contradictions is hampered profoundly by the tendency to reinterpret people's experiences in Western discursive forms. Spivak (1988) used the term 'ideological victimage' to express the disempowering effect of this tendency which is also described in several analyses of 'colonialist' discourse (for example, Chatterjee, 1986; Nandy, 1983; Wa Thiong'o, 1986; Said, 1978). Clearly one cannot see the world at all without the perceptual possibilities afforded by a linguistic and cultural tradition. However, the message for Westerners from these critiques is that this same linguistic and cultural tradition constitutes a blindfold as well – a blindfold which can be removed, but only partially removed, by thoughtful deference to the linguistic and cultural traditions of others.

This can only happen in concrete situations where people of different cultures come together to work on problems which in some way and in at least some part are seen to be of mutual concern and consequence. But how are we to set up the dialogical conditions which make these negotiations of meaning possible?

THE STORY BEGINS

One afternoon in 1989, Dr Alex Boyd, an Australian Health Action Associates community medicine specialist, practitioner and researcher who was working in the Sudan arrived at Deakin University in Geelong. She was seeking support for a community-based medical education program she planned to conduct for 'traditional birth attendants' in the Sudan. She came to Deakin because she had heard that in recent times the Deakin Action Research Group had turned its attention to the problems of conducting action research in cross-cultural contexts, especially in Aboriginal education. The theoretical and practical accomplishments of those monocultural and cross-cultural enquiries had become widely known. The Deakin participatory action research programme had developed extensive international venues for its publications (for example, Carr and Kemmis, 1986; Kemmis and McTaggart, 1988a, 1988b) and was also represented in various international forums (McTaggart, 1989a, 1989b). Of particular relevance was the movement of action research away from its conceptualization in terms of ideal images such as 'empowerment' or as collections of techniques, and towards culturally embracing notions which recognize the political economy of the research act in concrete engagement in a social movement.

Dr Boyd wanted Deakin to collaborate in the study she proposed for these reasons. I was interested to participate because it seemed that Dr Boyd's project agenda explored further many issues which has arisen out of our work in Aboriginal communities in the Northern Territory of Australia. It seemed that the provision of 'aid' internationally generated many issues we had already begun to grapple with. Almost all forms of transnational aid or intranational assistance to indigenous people make an assumption that local participants will be able to utilize the content and processes of the support to continue the work when the temporary structures of support are removed. That is, aid projects tend to have an **educative** intent. But what kinds of pedagogies are employed, and how do they address the problem of the transfer of ownership of the aid project's substance to the people it is designed to help? What are the conditions which enable or frustrate people in their efforts to study and improve their own practices? These were questions I had worked on in different contexts for several years (McTaggart, 1989c, 1989d).

It was obvious that the provision of Australian aid to the Sudan and supporting Australian Aboriginal people in their efforts to develop 'Aboriginal pedagogies' was not a culturally neutral activity. Aid provision and the pedagogies it entails intersect with existing forms of organization, indigenous ways of working, the ways in which indigenous people and aid providers relate to each other and among themselves, and the ways in which the indigenous activity the aid seeks to improve is conceptualized. Aid only 'works' if it is locked into local culture in some way, but local culture is dynamic so the very presence of aid affects local practices. I simply note here that many authors have argued that aid almost never 'works' and worse than that, has actually been extremely harmful in the Third World. I have identified these arguments elsewhere in an attempt to persuade Australian educators not to succumb to the exhortations of inter-national economic rationalism (McTaggart, 1992). For my current purpose, I want to regard the effects of aid practice as an **issue**, rather than as an inevitable failure.

Because the provision of aid affects local forms of life and work it sits on the horns of a dilemma. On one side is the trap of assuming that 'Western' solutions can simply be transplanted into other cultural settings, on the other is the prospect of the distortion of aid provi-sion in ways which actually make it counterproductive. Aid may be culturally destructive, or it may be destroyed itself, which, in terms of helping the people it is intended to help, amounts to the same thing.

In short, unless the practice of most aid provision is understood at the very least as a culturally sensitive **pedagogical** process, there are dangers that aid can be diverted away from, and perhaps even directed against the social purposes for which it was intended. That risk applies across all kinds of aid, for example, medical, educational and agricultural, because each has an impact on existing cultural processes. The risk may also be in evidence **within** each of these substantive areas to the nature of the initial proposal or request for aid, the actual con-tent of the aid, the processes by which it is realized, the implicit or explicit pedagogy by which understanding of the aid provision is created, and the methodologies by which it is evaluated and studied.

It seemed to me that any solution to the dilemma lies in establishing a mutually supportive dialectical relationship between particular aid projects and the cultures in which they are expected to exert their effects. It is clear that such relationships are very complex and likely to be quite site-specific. Nevertheless it seems possible that some general principles might be identified once actual practices are studied carefully. Who is helped, how, for how long, at what cost (economic and other) are important issues, but they are probably not as important as the nature and ultimate ownership of the expertise participation in the aid project fosters. Underlying all of these, what counts as legitimate knowledge of the world is at stake. Aid provision both initiates and confirms contestation about how the world is to be understood (and acted upon) – especially contestation between Western scientific knowledge (natural and social) which vindicates the legitimacy of the aid in Western terms and the popular knowledge of the people aid is meant to assist. Popular knowledge is all too easily delegitimated in post-colonial contexts where institutional knowledge (of medicine, for example) slips in on the coat-tails of colonial institutional hegemony (Nandy, 1983; Spivak, 1988).

Unless aid informs popular knowledge in acceptable ways, ways which actually sustain, strengthen and enrich the cultural practice of those it is meant to help, it may nurture dependence on outsiders and worsen disadvantage relative to other insiders. This raises two questions. How can we invent different pedagogies to respond to these issues? And, on the basis of the practical understandings and theoretical resources about pedagogy currently at our disposal, what are the possible options for the pedagogy of aid provision in the future? These were the questions which enticed me to accept Alex Boyd's invitation.

There seemed to me to be three research outcomes possible from participating. First, we could articulate a richer understanding of Australian aid provision theory and practice, especially of the ways in which indigenous people's views, culture and specific practices might be taken into account. I thought we might pay explicit attention to emergent concerns in the action research field, for example, the engagement of local knowledge, the relationship between research and social movements, and the practice of 'emancipation'. Second, and from a similar perspective, I thought we could critique our own project which had the explicit aim of training 'Traditional Birth Attendants' in Northern Sudan to adopt and adapt in 'culturally appropriate' ways Western birthing practices thought to improve infant and maternal post-natal health using a participatory action research approach. A third aim seemed to me to be to secure a new location for participatory action research as the convergence of the two intellectual traditions which informed and shaped what are known as 'action research' and 'participatory research'.

I thought five key bodies of literature could be drawn upon to inform the study: the theoretical rationale for action research (for example, Carr and Kemmis, 1986; Kemmis and McTaggart, 1988a, 1988b); the development of cross-cultural action research (McTaggart, 1991; Fals Borda, 1979; Freire, 1974, 1982); the participatory research tradition (Hall, 1979, 1982; Tandon, 1988); theories of the colonization of consciousness (Berger, Berger and Kellner, 1979; Wa Thiong'o, 1986;

Chatterjee, 1986; El Saadawi, 1980; Nandy, 1983; Spivak, 1988); and the critiques of Western approaches to aid and development themselves (Amin, 1990; Bello and Rosenfeld, 1990; Clark, 1991; George, 1988; Hancock, 1989; Hayter, 1981; Merchant, 1980; Rothbard, 1988; Shiva, 1989; Trainer, 1985, 1989; Tomlinson, 1991; Waring, 1988).

I thought that the project could be significant in several ways. First, it could take a unique perspective on aid projects by focusing on pedagogical aspects and could contribute to the theory underlying the ways in which aid projects are justified and the issues associated with them are understood. Second, it could help to make the practice of aid provision more effective by articulating a theoretically and practically informed approach to pedagogy and its results, increasing the likelihood that temporary ways of working within the aid project can be made more resilient as aid support is removed. Third, it could describe ways in which indigenous people contributed to the design, realization and evaluation of the project designed to assist them, and the kinds of effects this participation produced. Fourth, it could identify ways in which the transfer to indigenous people of the responsibility for work initiated in aid projects could be accomplished. Fifth, it could describe the strategies which were used to help to ensure that aid remains focused on those people in most need. Sixth, it could identify ways in which 'Western' solutions were remade by indigenous people for their own purposes and contexts to increase the sensitivity of pedagogies to the inevitability and potential of such outcomes.

My experience of working with traditionally oriented Aboriginal people in Australia had already taught me that it is easy to underestimate the complexity of the issues involved in work of this kind, and to overestimate the practical effects one project might have. Nevertheless, I thought it might be possible to articulate the issues themselves and agreed to seek support for the study from the Women in Development Fund (through the Australian International Development Assistance Bureau). Some time later I also sought related support from the Australian Research Council. I did not realize how many issues would lurch into existence even before the project began.

ISSUE 1: ON BEING 'WESTERN'

In our work with Aboriginal people I had consistently been reminded of the 'Westernness' of the content of our ideas, and of our pedagogy. Western 'education' has been a mixed blessing to other world cultures, sometimes proving more insidious and oppressive than the military conquests which preceded it. African Ngugi Wa Thiong'o, in describing the effects of Western education, put it most eloquently:

The night of the sword and the bullet was followed by the morning of the chalk and the blackboard . . . Real power resided not at all in the cannons of the first morning but in what followed . . . The new school had the nature of both the cannon and the magnet. From the cannon it took the efficiency of a fighting weapon. But better than the cannon it made the conquest permanent. The cannon forces the body and the school fascinates the soul (Wa Thiong'o, 1986)

Aboriginal writers in Australia have expressed similar reservations about the provision of education to their people. Wesley Lanhupuy, Member for Arnhem in the Northern Territory Legislative Assembly outlined the continuity between colonization and assimilation in Aboriginal education:

Schools have been part of the process of the colonization of Australia and its original inhabitants. This colonization process has taken place within living memory in the Northern Territory and unfortunately continues in many of our schools today. These have been difficult times, in which schools have been used quite openly to capture the minds of Aboriginal children and to turn them towards the dominant Balanda [Western] culture. So schools have been most significant in the attempt by non-Aboriginal Australians to assimilate Aborigines into the Balanda society . . . The strong Balanda cultural orientation of the [school] and the dominating position of Balanda teachers and administrators inevitably work to influence the minds of children in ways that undervalue the Aboriginal heritage. Aboriginal people now understand that if schools are to serve the political social and economic purposes of their own people, the school, as an institution, needs to be accommodated within Aboriginal society itself. Only when the cultural orientation of the school becomes Yolngu [Aboriginal] will schools become integral to the movement of Aborigines toward self-determination. The decolonization of schools in Aboriginal communities is the challenge for Aborigines now (Lanhupuy, 1987).

The term 'Balanda' employed by Lanhupuy is used by the Aboriginal people of Northeast Arnhemland in the Northern Territory of Australia to designate any person of European extraction. It derives from the the 'Hollander' which came to the attention of Aboriginal people during hundreds of years of contact with Macassan trepang fishers who visited the shores of Northeast Arnhemland from Indonesia. Indonesia, of course, was colonized by the Dutch during this period. The extended contact with the Macassans shows the ease with which Australian Aboriginal people can engage people and customs from some other cultures. That engagement includes recognizing and strengthening a sense of distinctive identity.

Aboriginal people have often been quite explicit about refusing to submit to Western ways of doing things. Aboriginal school principal (and lead singer of the band *Yothu-yindi*) Mandawuy Yunupingu explained:

> An appropriate curriculum for Yolngu is one that is located in the Aboriginal world which can enable the children to cross over to the Balanda world, the Ganma curriculum allows for identification of bits of Balanda knowledge that are consistent with the Yolngu way of learning. Yolngu learn their foundations (djalkiri) from their parents and relations – around them the learning occurs at home and in different ceremonies (Yunupingu, 1988a).

The term *Ganma* designates a very powerful and important concept in Yolngu Matha, the language(s) of the people of Northeast Arnhemland. It cannot be used by Aboriginal people without explicit permission from the most senior councils of their communities. Our understanding of it can never be complete, but Ganma refers to the way in which like and unlike are reconciled within Aboriginal culture (for example, in moiety-like relationships). Other Aboriginal teachers from Yunupingu's Yirrkala community described the concept of Ganma as it was interpreted for the Ganma Project, an attempt to negotiate Balanda and Yolngu meanings in education:

> In terms of the Ganma project, ganma is taken as desciding the situation where a river of water from the sea (in this case Balanda knowledge) and a river of water from the land (Yolngu knowledge) mutually engulf each other on flowing into a common lagoon and become one. In coming together the streams of water mix across the interface of the two currents and foam is created at the surface so that the process of ganma is marked by lines of foam along the interface of the two currents. In the terms of the metaphor, then the line of foam that is formed by the interaction of the two currents marks the interface between the current of Yolngu life and the current of Balanda life. Both Yolngu and Balanda can benefit from theorising over the interaction between two streams of life. This process of making knowledge of one world available in another is a familiar practice for us. Our world exists in two parts: the Dhuwa and the Yirritja. Dhuwa rom (knowledge of Dhuwa clans) is made available to Yirritja clans for their use and vice versa (Marika, Ngurruwutthun and White, 1992).

This kind of reconciliation is never easy. Tiwi (Aboriginal) teacher Wangintawujimawu (Wanginti) Tungutalum from Nguiu (Bathurst Island, north of Australia) explained the alienating effect of Westernism and the resolution of that tension in this way:

> Through my long experience as a Tiwi teacher, I have done everything I could to be more like a Non-Tiwi teacher (Murruntaka) . . . I have taught my Tiwi children using the concepts of Western styles of teaching. Tiwi children responded in so-called Western learning styles. I had not realised that the children were developing Western ways of learning, and becoming more Westernised. I have always felt a real tension between myself as a Tiwi woman, and the pressure to teach like Murrantawi. I now know what to do, I want my teaching, the curriculum and the school to become truly Tiwi . . . The development of a Tiwi Pedagogy will mean that the school is no longer an agent of cultural oppression and that Tiwi culture remains ours for me and my Tiwi people (Tungutalum, 1990).

These comments about one substantive area, education, are presented to indicate one, perhaps optimal, sense in which non-Westerners might make use of the resources of Westernism for their own purposes. But people are not always so aware nor sensitive to their own needs and desires to ensure the retention of a sense of cultural and personal identity. Their self-understandings leave them in a position which causes others concern and which might cause them concern if other perspectives were drawn to their attention. Alternatively, their self-understandings are sound enough, but they are in a weak and vulnerable position as far as taking ameliorative concrete action is concerned. How was the pedagogy of aid projects to be constituted in such situation?

ISSUE 2: BIRTH AND HEALTH IN THE SUDAN

I knew a little about the practice of 'female circumcision' in Africa when Alex Boyd came to my office that afternoon, but I did not know then that my subsequent reading would create such a conflict between my respect for cultural relativism and my views about social justice. The position of women in the Sudan raises these issues in a very unpleasant way. Traditional Birth Attendants, for whom we planned to design and conduct 'training' workshops, were responsible not only for midwifery practices, but also for the practice of circumcision. The practice has a serious effect on the health of both women and female children. I was shocked by the severity and extent of the practice: female circumcision is widely practised and the results adversely affect the health of women at all times but especially during and after childbirth. Infant mortality and morbidity were also increased substantially by the practice. The practice varies in nature and intensity throughout the Sudan, but El Saadawi described a typical example in these terms:

> The clitoris, external lips and internal lips are completely excised, and the orifice and the genital organs closed with a flap of sheep's intestines leaving only a very small opening barely sufficient to let the tip of the finger in, so that menstrual and urinary flows are not held back. This opening is slit at the time of marriage and widened to allow penetration of the male sexual organ. It is widened again when a child is born and then narrowed down once more. Complete closure of the aperture is also done on a woman who is divorced, so that she literally becomes a virgin once more and can have no sexual intercourse except in the eventuality of marriage, in which case the opening is restored (El Saadawi, 1980).

Though Western medical practice may have an undistinguished record in its treatment of Western women, it would call such practices into question (leaving aside other grounds obvious to Westerners). Naming the practice itself was an issue. Some feminists prefer the term 'clitoridectomy' (Spivak, 1988), but in the Sudanese case this is an anatomical understatement of seriously misleading degree. In the past few years Western feminists, especially those familiar with its more extreme forms, have been adamant that the practice should be called 'genital mutilation', a term I thought was appropriate myself. But Alex Boyd and others (Lightfoot-Klein, 1989) were less sure that this was appropriate. Despite the fact that the practice had been made illegal by a liberal government in the Sudan, the term used for the practice by Sudanese women was the term for circumcision, exactly the same word as was used for male circumcision.

Helping Sudanese women to confront the suffering caused by this brutal, but widely accepted practice, was not likely to be easy, despite its illegality. El Saadawi attributed this difficulty to a deeply entrenched patriarchal economic system which was actually made more virulently oppressive by the responses of Islam to the excesses of Western colonialism:

> The thousands of *dayas*, nurses, para-medical staff and doctors who make money out of female circumcision, naturally resist any change in these values and practices which are a source of gain to them. In the Sudan there is a veritable army of *dayas* who earn a livelihood out of the series of operations performed on women, either to excise their external genital organs, or to narrow and widen the outer aperture according to whether a woman is

marrying, divorcing, remarrying, having a child or recovering from labour (El Saadawi, 1980).

The *dayas*, or Traditional Birth Attendants, were also responsible for the initial circumcision and infibulation of young girls in the Sudan, usually between the ages of four and eight, but sometimes as early as two and as late as eleven years of age (Lightfoot-Klein, 1989).

My first impulse in these early discussions about how we might work was to call upon medical evidence to show the relationship between mortality and severity of excision – to begin to create a pedagogy which might increase the probability that women were less victimized by the coalescence of the religious, medical and economic systems they find themselves in. It seemed to me that workshop participants themselves **might** come to regard the differences evident in each village as an issue, even if it was not something which was spontaneously identified as such in the workshops Dr Boyd was to conduct with them. But what if they did not? How did the women see themselves? Were they Muslim first and women second? Were they Sudanese persons before they were (medical) bodies? What **was** the relationship between a particular woman's gender and her ethnicity? Tsolidis (1986) indicated that such tensions are deeply socially constructed. Longstanding practices seemed unlikely to bend to the balmy breeze of any outsider's good idea.

I knew that we should elect to take a participatory action research approach which encouraged people to document and reflect upon current practices, the discourses which help constitute and describe them, and the forms of social organization and power relationships these entail. In Freire's terms:

I must try . . . to have the people dialogically involved as . . . researchers with me. If I am interested in knowing the people's ways of thinking and levels of perception, then the people have to think about their thinking and not be only the objects of my thinking. This method of investigation which involves study – and criticism of the study – by people is at the same time a learning process. Through this process of investigation, examination, criticism and reinvestigation, the level of critical thinking is raised among all those involved (Freire, 1982).

That is, I thought that the theory and practice of both community health **and** participatory action research itself could be subjected to critique directly by all participants at all levels, birthing mothers, birth attendants, community health and community education workers, central hospital staff and academics. But I knew that even this strategy did not ensure that participants' interests would be completely protected. From Said's (1978) account of 'orientalism' in Muslim contexts two points could be made: first, our own cultural hegemony is such that we may be deceiving ourselves, and second, the people themselves may also be so deceived for related reasons. Nevertheless, when asked to help we could see no alternative to trying to maintain the dialogue and being vigilant about the way hegemony works. I thought the ways in which those mutually confirming deceptions are confirmed and confronted could constitute an important theoretical focus of the study.

ISSUE 3: WAS THE STUDY 'DO-ABLE'?

The study I envisaged would employ the methodology of participatory action research. But I thought that the cultural context would necessitate a much stronger commitment to a phenomenological understanding using the standard approaches to interpretive enquiry, interview (especially), observation and document analysis with considerable help from bilingual Sudanese. This dependence in itself was an issue. I had no Arabic myself, Alex Boyd had only a little, and as in most Third World contexts, the people most likely to speak English were those who had experienced an English education, often only accessible to already advantaged social groups.

This concern was sharpened by direct experience. In our work with Aboriginal people, it often seemed that our efforts were appreciated and certainly preferred over other Western efforts in several communities, but our own monolingualism meant that testimony to that effect came almost exclusively from bilingual Aboriginal people. We disciplined our work with one question foremost in our minds: 'Were we the best friends or worst enemies of the Aboriginal people who entrusted us with requests for support?' It was a salutory experience for us to find that the Aboriginal teachers with whom we worked addressed the same question to themselves about their relationships with other Aboriginal people in their communities. It is not easy to find any real comfort about one's own authenticity in such circumstances. Of course, the commitment to maintain dialogue around the issue is the best one can do once the decision to do anything is made, but it is not a simple remedy for an easy conscience.

I knew that in the Sudan the sources of understanding would be participants in the Traditional Birth Attendant training programme, that is, community health field workers who were adapting their own practices to make them more sensitive to, and supportive of, their 'clients'. Data collection to inform my own action research would have to be conducted primarily through Dr Alexandra Boyd's staff because of language difficulties and Muslim prohibitions. These health workers were attached to central hospitals (Khartoum and Omdurman) and to local communities. But I did not have much sense of the politics of these relationships, and even though I had spent a fairly intensive afternoon with Alex Boyd, I did not know where she stood (or at least where she was **seen** to stand) in the local political scene. My experience in Aboriginal communities (as well as in a variety of evaluation studies and contexts) indicated that just who introduced me was a very important determinant of the kinds of relationships which were possible for a very long time. I was worried about whether I could do anything useful at all, and raised the question about the worth of investing a substantial sum of money in yet another Western middle class male academic who happened to have written a little about action research in other contexts.

ISSUE 4: LEGITIMATION?

Alex Boyd thought that these concerns could be addressed. She argued that my involvement was justified in several different ways. First, the fact that I had been involved in the publication of several books and articles about action research would help to legitimate the work in communities in which she (and other local people) had already begun. Second, the way in which room could be created for the work to continue would be to have a white male academic to help mount the case for it in the patriarchal academic and policy formation establishment. It was thought that a male academic could do more to persuade other male members of the predominantly male medical, academic and bureaucratic institutional and perhaps even local contexts of reform that participatory action research was an appropriate alternative to the standardized application of Western medical solutions. In one sense, it was not so much the content of the publications which might be useful, but that such work existed at all. This had certainly appeared to be the case in other contexts in which I had worked. Documentation was less important substantively, people had their own well-tested ideas. But institutional legitimation helped in the *realpolitik* of a particular social context.

Of course, such legitimation is a two-edged sword. Efforts to develop distinctive modes of discourse, social relationships (and organization) and practice which might 'define' action research were always prone to accusations of exclusivity and academic imperialism, especially from the advocates of participatory research and popular knowledge (Chaudhary, forthcoming; Fals Borda and Rahman, 1991). Why should people do 'participatory action research' as **we** understood it? Of course, we could aspire to learn from each other and to achieve reciprocity and symmetry in our ways of working and talking together, but how might we negotiate and judge that in a cross-cultural situation?

Even in Western social science there are important issues to engage about the sheer possibility of reciprocity and symmetry in discursive relations. In the literature of critical theory, there is a somewhat contested aspiration underlying each of these concepts – the ideal of 'symmetrial communication' which derives from Jürgen Habermas' conceptualization of an 'ideal speech situation' (Kemmis, 1980: Carr and Kemmis, 1986). It means the use of discourse to attempt 'to come to an agreement about the truth of a problematic statement or the correctness of a problematic norm and carries with it a supposition that a genuine agreement is possible'. Habermas argued that provided the 'rational' decision is based solely on better argument, such agreement is possible. The characteristic demanded of discussion to achieve this end is that it be 'free from all constraints of domination, whether their source be conscious strategic behaviour or communication barriers secured in ideology or neurosis'. 'In particular, all participants must have the same chance to initiate, and perpetuate discourse, to put forward, call into question, and give reasons for or against statements, explanations, interpretations and justifications. Furthermore, they must have the same chance to express attitudes, feelings, intentions and the like, and to command, to oppose, to permit, to forbid, etc.' (McCarthy, 1978, cited in McTaggart and Fitzpatrick, 1981).

The logical and practical possibilities of the 'ideal speech situation' where discourse is 'freed from the constraints of action' in the interests of the pursuit of truth have been challenged in several ways (Nielsen, 1983; Connolly, 1987). One cluster of criticism questions its fundamental consensualism, arguing instead that all aspects of speech are fundamentally contestable. Another related cluster of concern challenges the assumption that people will become committed to discourses which, through their symmetry, act against their own interests (throwing away the advantages they have achieved because of the inequities capitalism creates). However, it is important to recognize that the idea was presented by Habermas as a working proposition (and now seems to attach less importance to it). Nevertheless, there does not seem to me to be any other solution than a conscientious and informed effort to engage these issues with others in practical situations on concrete tasks where language, social relationships and activities are jointly scrutinized for their implicit and explicit politics. That is, if the issue is engaged concretely, the validity of the premised ideal speech situation is somewhat beside the point.

Still, the aspiration to help people to see their worlds more clearly, or even just somewhat differently, is difficult enough in Western, supposedly monocultural contexts. Just think, for example, of the allegations of pomposity directed at Marxist notions of 'false' or 'distorted' consciousness, not to mention the gender blindness of historical and dialectical materialism in spite of their emancipatory aspirations.

ISSUE 5: WHITE KNIGHTS AND WESTERN FEMINISM

It seemed clear to me that there were many things a participatory action research project with Traditional Birth Attendants might achieve even if the issue of genital mutilation was not engaged. The social role of the TBAs made them important arbiters of 'medical' knowledge, and in situations where health is often seriously threatened by elementary things such as insanitary water, much could be done to exploit and coopt Western understandings in ways that Sudanese women found appropriate to them. But I could not bring myself to ignore what to me seemed like unforgivable butchery to achieve some partiarchally imposed ideal. Its effects on health (in my definition) were central, even if the social justice could be left aside.

But how could it be any of my business anyway? Did my own gender(ing) mean that I could not come to understand the nature of the issue in ways which helped women to protect themselves from the patriarchal virginity cult, which, in my eyes, made them victims. Could I honour aspirations expressed by Elizabeth Grosz for feminist theory and practice?

> As a series of strategic interventions into patriarchal social and theoretical paradigms, feminism must develop a versatile and wide-ranging set of conceptual tools and methodological procedures to arm itself defensively and offensively. It requires weapons to challenge patriarchal intellectual norms; and by which to protect itself against various counter-attacks from the existing regimes of power. Feminists can ignore history and current conceptions of theories of human subjectivity only at their own peril. Feminist theory need not commit itself to the values and assumptions governing patriarchal knowledges; but in order to go *beyond* them, it must work through them, understand them, displace them in order to create a space of its own, a space designed and inhabited by women, capable of expressing their interests and values (Grosz, 1990).

Despite the separatist tone of the later phrasing, it did not seem to me impossible to make a contribution to this analysis of patriarchy. I did not think that such a 'space of its own' excluded the possibility of male participation. Indeed, such space might be just as desirable to (some) men as it was for women. Participatory action research belonged to a tradition which confronted hierarchical arrangements, mostly Western and patriarchal, so I could see some potential for productive work and learning. The participatory research movement itself had been informed by the efforts of many women activists in the Third World (Shiva, 1989; Chen, 1983; Bhasin, 1978; Fals Borda and Rahman, 1991). Furthermore, Western and academic feminists themselves were reminded by Spivak that their own theory and methodology needed to be conscious of the highly differentiated forms of feminism in the Third World. Referring to the lives of two illiterate Indian women trapped in a colonized view of self and land she wrote:

> I should not consequently patronize these women, not yet enter-
> tain a nostalgia for being as they are. The academic feminist must
> learn to learn from them, to speak to them, to suspect that their
> access to the political and sexual scene is not merely to be *corrected*
> by our superior theory and enlightened compassion. Is our
> insistence on the beauty of the old necessarily to be preferred
> to a careless acknowledgement of the mutability of sexuality?
> What of the fact that my distance from those two was, however
> micrologically you defined class, class-determined and
> determining?
>
> How, then, can one learn from and speak to the millions of
> illiterate rural and urban Indian women who live 'in the pores
> of' capitalism, inaccessible to the capitalist dynamics that allow
> us shared channels of communication, the definition of common
> enemies? The pioneering books that bring First World feminists
> news from the Third World are written by privileged informants
> and can only be deciphered by a trained readership. The distance
> between 'the informant's world,' 'her own sense of the world
> she writes about,' and that of the non-specialist feminist is so
> great that, paradoxically, *pace* the subtleties of reader-response
> theories, here the distinctions might be missed.
>
> This is not the tired nationalist claim that only a native
> can know the scene. The point that I am trying to make is
> that, in order to learn enough about Third World women and
> to develop a different readership, the immense heterogeneity
> of the field must be appreciated, and the First World feminist
> must learn to stop feeling privileged *as a woman* (Spivak, 1988).

The point about diversity is important, but is not conceptualization of the relationship between First World and Third World women here an issue in another sense? How are Third World women to be learned about, and is their relationship with the First World to be as a 'reader-ship'? Is that the way they are best supported by First World women?

Clearly there is much in Western feminist theory (and in other bodies of knowledge) which is potentially useful to Third World women. But how is support for their efforts to be given expression? Potentially at least, participatory action research seemed to me to a very effective way likely to be more effective than an exegesis of Third World texts and relationships forged around an anticipation of 'readership'. Perhaps I could learn more by direct experience. At the very least, I could learn in more significant ways that personal engagement at the site was not likely to be effective.

From the texts produced about the Sudan, I knew that the practice of genital mutilation and its results were highly valued by women, a hallmark of beauty, of course a beauty defined long ago in terms which meant attractiveness to men as unspoiled chattles. Unfortunately, girls whose middle class parents opted for a milder form of mutilation (usually in the cities) sometimes found that grandmothers secretly took the girls away to a more traditional *daya* for more severe treatment. Their aim was to protect the attractiveness and marriage-worthiness of the young girl. In short, in their view, the child was being done a favour.

I was even more moved to participate when I discovered that the matter was as much to do with the rights of children. Lightfoot-Klein (1989) cited the work of McLean (1980) to illustrate the sheer brutality of the typical procedure. The example occurred at Djibouti near the eastern Sudanese border:

> The little girl, entirely nude, is immobilized in the sitting position on a low stool by at least three women. One of them with her arms tightly around the little girl's chest; two others hold the child's thighs apart by force, in order to open wide the vulva. The child's arms are tied behind her back, or immobilized by two other women guests. The traditional operator says a short prayer: 'Allah is great and Mohammed is his prophet. May Allah keep away all evils.' Then she spreads on the floor some offerings to Allah: split maize, or, in urban areas, eggs. Then the old woman takes out her razor and excises the clitoris. The infibulation follows: the operator cuts with her razor from top to bottom of the small lip and scrapes the flesh from the inside of the large lip. This nymphectomy and scraping are repeated on the other side of the vulva. The little girl howls and writhes in pain, although strongly held down. The operator wipes the blood from the wound, and the mother, as well as the guests, 'verify' her work, sometimes putting their fingers in. The amount of scraping of the large lips depends in the 'technical' ability of the operator. The opening left for urine and menstrual blood is miniscule. Then the operator applies a paste and ensures the adhesion of the large

lips by means of an acacia thorn, which pierces one lip and passes through into the other. She sticks in three or four in this manner down the vulva. These thorns are held in place either by means of sewing thread or with horsehair. Paste is again put on the wound. But all this is not sufficient to ensure coalescence of the large lips, so the little girl is then tied up from her pelvis to her feet; strips of material rolled up into rope immobilize her legs entirely. Exhausted, the little girl is then dressed and put on a bed. The operation lasts from fifteen to twenty minutes according to the ability of the old woman and the resistance put up by the child (McLean, 1980, cited in Lightfoot-Klein, 1989).

One contribution which has been made to this practice has been the availability of anaesthesia. According to Lightfoot-Klein this has served to **increase** the severity of the practice by reducing the pain and the propensity of the child to resist. This contribution of Western medicine could hardly be viewed as a success – in Western terms. How Western ideas might be utilized in the Sudan was an issue with serious practical as well as cultural and ideological implications.

Though there is a reference to Allah in the traditional operator's prayer in the quote above, some authors have argued that this should not be taken to mean that the practice is encouraged or endorsed in the Koran. They report that it is not mentioned. Lightfoot-Klein (1989) and El Saadawi (1980) contest the assumption that is sometimes made that genital mutilation is an edict of Islam. An appeal attributed to the Prophet Mohammed for moderation of the practice in some texts is interpreted by these authors as a rejection of it rather than as endorsement as some suppose. But Assad (1980, cited in Lightfoot-Klein, 1989) noted that the official position of Islamic jurists in the countries that practise it is as follows:

> Female circumcision is an Islamic tradition mentioned in the tradition of the Prophet, and sanctioned by the Imams [religious leaders] and Jurists in spite of their differences on whether it is duty of *Sunna* [tradition]. We support the practice and sanction it in view of its effect on attenuating the sexual desire of women and directing it to desirable moderation.

Despite this position, it is worth noting also that the practice predates both Islam and Christianity by thousands of years. The difficulty of reconciling these different interpretations is one of the key problems in working cross-culturally. But how does one engage the difficulty?

I was persuaded that sitting at my desk was a less moral course of action than trying to do **something**. The next challenge I confronted was 'Why do something about the patriarchy in the Sudan, when it was so evident in me and all around me?' It was easy to say that I had been 'invited' to participate in the Sudan and that that ended the moral dilemma about how I might spend my time. It would have been even easier to rationalize my position by saying to myself that I was doing something for gender equity in my own cultural context because I happened to be working on a case study of gender issues in a co-educational private school at that time.

I thought at first that the female genital mutilation issue was distinctively African and to a lesser degree Middle Eastern. The practice has been in evidence in some non-Western Australian communities, but was relatively uncommon, and generally less severe than the example I have described. Though clitoridectomy or more extensive mutilation would not be viewed as an acceptable practice by most conventional Australian moral or legal standards, the issue has not received much attention. It would be a profound test of the Australian government's explicit commitment to 'multiculturalism' on the one hand and gender equity on the other. For ordinary cultural reasons as much as any other, the practice is well-hidden. This obviously makes it difficult to assess extent and severity in this Western context, and there was little chance that I would be invited to do anything about women's health as I had been in the Sudan. Besides, oppression can be either concrete or hegemonic, and it was obvious that the suppression and redirection of female sexuality was also a significant preoccupation of Westernism, and among Australians themselves. The punitive orientation of patriarchal ideology and institutions in matters of female sexuality was patently evident (Spivak, 1988; MacKinnon, 1989). The very conceptualizations of sexuality for women are in terms of species reproduction on the one hand and the pleasures of men on the other (rather than pleasure for women, or at least pleasure of a somewhat momentary kind). This was evident at several levels.

How could one say that the mutilation of women in the Sudan differed in principle from the Western patriarchally inspired practices of (i) the 'improvement' of women's bodies by means of medically unnecessary 'cosmetic' surgery and dieting, (ii) the distortion of women's feet and posture by inappropriate footwear, (iii) the insidious poisoning of women from silicon leakage from artificial breast implantation, (iv) the excessive use of hysterectomy as a means of mediating the onset of menopause, (v) the experimentation with women's bodies implicit in chemical birth control, stimulation of fertility, and in the biochemical support applied during artificial insemination by donor (Rowland, 1991). It is obviously not possible here to justify or even to catalogue the effects of male hegemony on the physical well-being of women's bodies. I identify these merely as examples and do not suggest that this encapsulates the effects of male hegemony.

Lest anyone should think that I am suggesting that these activities occur without the 'consent' of the women involved, I say simply that it is obvious that consent is typically obtained in the cases I have identified. Indeed, many of the physical invasions are actively sought by women. This signifies nothing more than the fact that hegemony has a perverse effect – it creates the illusion of consent. Of course, consent is always situational; it is a choice among known options. When options do not include or allow the imagination of alternatives, consent to abuse of some kind is merely the selection of one inappropriate alternative ahead of others (if indeed any others are known). Gramsci has argued that hegemony is never complete, but these examples suggest it comes close. However, male domination and violation of women's bodies in Western contexts is not simply left to hegemony, it is often concrete and protected after the event by a complex of male-dominated institutional arrangements (MacKinnon, 1989). In both the West and the Third World, phallocentric hegemony was evident, for example, in the persistent naming of female mutilation as 'circumcision', the same term generally applied to the removal of a small amount of the prepuce with absolutely no effect on function, health or pleasure in the male.

Should I spend my time on gender issues (or indeed on other issues altogether) in my own culture rather than in the Sudan? Of course, it was obvious that I should do both (recognizing that only an Occidental would lapse into such dualism). I elected to take the opportunity to visit the Sudan to work with Alex Boyd, at the very least to inform a future decision about what it might be possible to accomplish. I do not deny that there was a certain fascination for me in travelling to the East: I cannot pretend that the excitement, adventure, gendering and enculturation of the pith helmet odysseys of the *Boys' Own Annual* genre I read with fervour in my youth left me unaffected. But I believe that I made a reasonable assessment, and it did seem to me that the invitation to participate came from someone with a better-grounded sense of what it was appropriate to do.

By telex, I indicated to the faculty members from the University of Khartoum who were to collaborate on the project that I preferred that women's groups concerned about the practice of circumcision were involved in the workshop. I had discussed this with Alex Boyd when she visited Australia and we decided that it was an appropriate course of action, but as a strategic issue we were not sure that this was the appropriate way of proceeding. Nevertheless, the suggestion was apparently agreeable to the Sudanese, and as I made my travel arrangements I understood that they had begun to organize a visa for me. It was obviously going to be important for men to be involved in discussion of these issues, but it seemed unlikely that it could or even should happen early, and the logistics alone made it a lower priority. Many telex and fax messages changed hands (or failed to arrive) and it seemed that a visa would never be forthcoming.

During the eighteen months of preparation and delay, the government of the Sudan changed. I was informed that a group of young Muslim military officers had taken over, and had committed the Sudanese people to more strict observance of *shari'a* (divine law). Among other things, this meant a change in the way in which rights in the Sudan were gendered if we can extrapolate from experience in other Muslim countries (Mernissi, 1987). Further, the change in government led to a chain of events which, in summary, meant that Westernism was more generally frowned upon, Alexandra Boyd's visa status became quite uncertain, the people in the university of Khartoum with whom we were to work changed roles within the university, and this in turn, meant that their participation in the TBA training curriculum development became impossible. I made arrangements on three occasions to go to the Sudan; each time I awaited a visa number in vain. I set myself a final deadline during 1990 for the cancellation of my third set of arrangements if a visa number was not relayed to me. On the day of my deadline, the Iraqi army invaded Kuwait.

As I watched television that night wondering how events might have appeared had I been in Khartoum, Egyptian political commentators were interviewed on the balcony of the Meridien Hotel in Cairo, overlooking the Nile. That hotel was where I had planned to stay prior to meeting two medical anthropologists from the United States on my way to the Sudan. I could not help feeling a many-faceted relief.

AFTERWORD: BROADENING THE FOCUS AND REDIRECTING THE LENS

In retrospect, it may appear that I have focused too much on the one issue of genital mutilation. I apologize for that, but think that it throws up some of the most important issues in cross-cultural contact. For a start, my emphasis reflects the emphasis in the literature I had access to. That emphasis itself demonstrates an aspect of the attitude of Occidental to Oriental. The focus is often on the unpleasant. Nevertheless, an anathema so self-evident to Westerners brings into sharp focus the tendency to Western cultural imperialism on the one hand and the commitments of the West to certain practices of social justice on the other.

But if it is so easy to see fault in others, perhaps it is because we do not spend enough time looking for it within our own cultural context. The narrowness of the focus taken in thinking about the project simply raises broader issues for me again. The experience crystallized concerns I have had about Western cultural imperialism (McTaggart, 1991b) in Aboriginal Australia and expressions of that same cultural imperialism in the provision of aid to the Third World and in Western conceptualizations of development. We ought to be concerned about the migration of unfettered neo-capitalism into cultures which may not have the discourses, social organization or institutionalized practices of resistance which have developed in Western nations. But these concerns ought also to lead us back to expressions of modern capitalism in our own institutional cultures.

Because of my work in programme evaluation in particular, I have been led to think more carefully about the ways in which we conceptualize accountability (McTaggart, 1988). During the 1980s, I was worried about the effects of 'corporate managerialism' as it was expressed in the 'restructuring' of state education ministries. In retrospect, that restructuring looks like cultural imperialism too, the imposition of an ideology of control which contested educators' ways of discussing their work. I am older, wiser and still much alarmed because the nationalization of the Australian curriculum places us in the grip of a discourse and politics of accountability which we should call into serious question. To identify the problem we confront we need to see ourselves as participants in a new world economic order. By looking both outwards and inwards we can see that 'aid' and 'development' relationships between the West and the Third World both inform us and cause us to question our commitments to the most recent expressions of Westernism.

AID AND DEVELOPMENT IN THE THIRD WORLD

The devastating effect of most Western 'aid' in Third World contexts is alarming and well-documented (for example, Clarke, 1991; Hancock, 1989; Trainer, 1985, 1989; Amin, 1990; Merchant, 1980; Shiva, 1989; Hayter, 1981). It is also apparently ignored in many government and non-government organizations (NGOs). Aid and development practised by the West express an ideology which is economistic, patriarchal, individualistic, Judaeo-Christian and Western democratic (with a thoroughly misplaced optimism about the role of the state in many Third **and** First World contexts (Amin, 1990; MacKinnon, 1989). Moral idealism is subordinated to materialism. The cornerstone of this ideology is a persistent and unexamined confidence in Western economic systems (a particular species of economism) despite their demonstrable ecological unsustainability. It is now clear that proceeding as the West has done since the industrial revolution (or perhaps even since the 'West' itself began in Mesopotamia (Starhawk, 1987) leads inevitably to the death of the planet.

In **all** forms of social life, what we see globally is what we see locally: the emergence of a new fundamentalism, the search for profit hidden in the guise of rational economics as the new world science. It promises (rather than premises) a universal economic order of modernity, progress and development, a promise to free the world from poverty. The new 'economic rationalism' is a worldwide phenomenon which 'guides' not only the conduct of transnational corporations, but governments and their agencies as well. It does so with increasing efficacy and pervasiveness (Rothbard, 1988; Pusey, 1991). I use the term 'guides' here in quotes to make a particular point. Economic rationalism is not merely a term which suggests the primacy of economic values. It **expresses** commitment to those values in order to serve particular sets of interests ahead of others. Furthermore, it **disguises** that commitment in a discourse of 'economic necessity' defined by its economic models. We have moved beyond the reductionism which leads all questions to be discussed as if they were economic ones (de-valuation) to a situation where moral questions are denied completely (de-moralization) in a cult of economic inevitability (as if greed had nothing to do with it). Broudy (1981) has described 'de-valuation' and 'de-moralization' in the following way:

> De-valuation refers to diminishing or denying the relevance of all but one type of value to an issue; de-moralization denies the relevance of moral questions. The reduction of all values – intellectual, civic, health, among others – to a money value would be an example of de-valuation; the slogan 'business is business' is an example of de-moralization (Broudy, 1981).

A description of national economies judged to 'work' by some economists and interested others (even if they do not; see Bello and Rosenfeld (1990)) has been idealized as a series of models which in turn become a social, political and cultural prescription for the rest of the world. Thus, the commitment is not to a particular 'scientific' stance, but rather to the interests of certain dominant groups, the individuals who practise and benefit from worldwide corporate business. These interests are not readily visible because the discursive forms in which they are presented are designed to hide them. Indeed, in Australia, society itself can be seen by economic rationalists as an obstacle to the scientific perfection of their models:

> Since the 1970s, reality has been turned upside down and society has been cast as the object of politics (rather than, at least in the

norms of earlier discourses, as the subject of politics). Further, society has been represented as some sort of stubbornly resisting sludge, as a 'generic externality' and even as an idealized opponent of 'the economy' (Pusey, 1991).

From the 'development' and 'aid' literatures it is easy to provide a snapshot of the way certain sectional interests are served.

WESTERNISM IN THE WEST AND AMONG ITS CONVERTS

The post-modern expression of Westernism as internationalist economics (Hinkson, 1991) has its victims in the West, too. Britons (or at least some Britons) are victim to IMF and World Bank prescriptions of the 1970s. Some of the vaunted success stories of implementation of these prescriptions during the 1980s are also becoming somewhat tarnished. The new economic 'dragons', Taiwan, South Korea, and Singapore, are in trouble. The economic revolution which was built on the backs of exploited female labour confronts the slowing of growth, civil unrest as workers realize that they get little from the revolution, increasingly authoritarian regimes, declining markets, highly concentrated foreign ownership (by Japanese transnational corporations) and environmental devastation (Bello and Rosenfeld, 1990).

These prescriptions echo internally as the exhortations to Westernize (or more subtly to 'internationalize') reverberate around the world. Action researchers can help to resist those aspects of Westernism and those aspects of their own cultural condition which they find oppressive. But to be credible, action researchers need to work to improve the rationality, justice, coherence and satisfactoriness of practice in their own cultural contexts. Current economic ideology provides the socially aware with plenty of scope for concern. Economic rationalism at home embodies all that is ill about 'development' – it is economistic, patriarchal, individualistic, Judaeo-Christian and Western democratic with moral idealism subordinated to materialism. It creates social problems which signify a deep malaise we need to attend at home.

Nevertheless, we must continue to worry about oppression in its various guises in other cultures. The worst aspects of Westernism are evidently not the only source of oppression on the planet. At least when invited, as Kemmis (1992) has argued, we need to work practically and theoretically to help people to analyse their suffering (Fay, 1975; 1988), to articulate the conditions which disfigure their lives (Hall, 1986), and to use these processes of enlightenment to help develop social movements which can change the conditions of social life which maintain irrationality, injustice and incoherent and unsatisfying forms of existence.

REFERENCES

Amin, Samir (1990) *Maldevelopment: anatomy of a global failure*, United Nations Press, Tokyo; Zed, London.

Bello, W., and Rosenfeld, S. (1990) *Dragons in distress: Asia's miracle economies in crisis*, Institute for Food and Development Policy, San Francisco.

Berger, P., Berger, B., and Kellner, H. (1973) *The homeless mind: Modernization and consciousness*, Random House, New York.

Bhasin, K. (1978) *Breaking barriers: A south Asian experience*, FAO, Bangkok and Paris.

Broudy, H.S. (1981) *Truth and credibility*, Longman, New York.

Carr, W., and Kemmis, S. (1986) *Becoming critical: Education, knowledge and action research*, Falmer, London.

Chatterjee, P. (1986) *Nationalist thought and the colonial world*, Zed, London.

Chaudhary, A.K. (forthcoming) Towards an epistemology of participatory research, in *Participatory action research: Contexts and consequences* R. McTaggart (ed.).

Chen, M.A. (1983) *A quiet revolution: Women in transition in rural Bangladesh*, Schenkman, Cambridge MA.

Clark, J. (1991) *Democratizing development: The role of voluntary organizations*, Earthscan, London.

Connolly, W.E. (1987) *Politics and ambiguity*, University of Wisconsin Press, Madison WI.

El Saadawi, N. (1980) *The golden face of Eve: Women in the Arab world*, Zed, London.

Fals Borda, O. (1979) Investigating reality in order to change it: The Colombian experience. *Dialectical Anthropology*, **4**, 33–55.

Fals Borda, O., and Rahman, M.A. (1991) *Action and knowledge: Breaking the monopoly with participatory action research*, Apex, New York.

Fay, B. (1975) *Social theory and political practice*, George Allen and Unwin, London.

Fay, B. (1988) *Critical social science*, Cornell University Press, Ithaca, NY.

Fitzpatrick, M. and McTaggart, R. (1981, December) *The requirements of a successful action program*. Paper presented at the Annual Conference of the Australian Association for Research in Education, Sydney.

Foucault, M. (1973) *The order of things: An archaeology of the human sciences* (trans. A. Sheridan Smith), Tavistock, London.

Freire, P. (1974) Extension or communication (trans. L. Bigwood and M. Marshall), in P. Freire, *Education: The practice of freedom*, London Writers and Readers Publishing Cooperative, London pp. 91–162.

Freire, P. (1982) Creating alternative research methods: Learning to do it by doing it, in *Creating knowledge: A monopoly?* (eds. B. Hall, A. Gillette and R. Tandon), Society for Participatory Research in Asia, Khanpur, New Delhi pp. 29–37.

George, S. (1988) *A fate worse than debt*, Penguin, London.

Grosz, E. (1990) Contemporary theories of power and subjectivity, in *Feminist knowledge: Critique and construct*, S. Gunew (ed.), Routledge, London pp. 59–120.

Habermas, J. (1972) *Theory and practice* (trans. J.J. Shapiro), Heinemann, London.

Habermas, J. (1974) *Knowledge and human interest* (trans. J. Viertel), Heinemann, London.

Hall, B.L. (1979) Knowledge as a commodity and participatory research. *Prospects*, **9 (4)**, 393–408.

Hall, B.L. (1981) Participatory research, popular knowledge and power: A personal reflection. *Convergence*, **14 (3)**,6–19.

Hall, S. (1986) On postmodernism and articulation: An interview [by Lawrence Grossberg]. *Journal of Communication Inquiry*, **10 (2)**, 40–56.

Hancock, G. (1989) *Lords of poverty: The power, prestige, and corruption of the international aid business*, Atlantic Monthly and MacMillan, New York.

Hayter, T. (1981) *The creation of world poverty*, Pluto, London.

Hinkson, J.(1991) *Postmodernity: State and education*, Deakin University Press, Geelong, Australia.

Kemmis, S. (1980) Symmetrical communications: Developing mutual understanding and consensus in course teams, in *Evaluation and distance teaching* (eds. J.E. Armstrong and R. Store), Townsville College of Advanced Education, Townsville, Australia.

Kemmis, S. (1992, March) *Pratica de la teoria critica ensenanza: Experiencias*. Lectures given (in English) at an international symposium at the University of Valladolid, Spain.

Kemmis, S., and McTaggart, R. (eds.) (1988a) *The action research planner (3rd ed.)*, Deakin University Press, Geelong, Australia.

Kemmis, S., and McTaggart, R. (eds.) (1988b) *The action research reader (3rd ed.)*, Deakin University Press, Geelong, Australia.

Lanhupuy, W. (1987) Balanda education: A mixed blessing for Aborigines, *The Aboriginal Child at School*, **15 (3)**, 31–36.

Lightfoot-Klein, H. (1989) *Prisoners of ritual: An odyssey into female genital circumcision in Africa*, Harrington Park, Binghamton NY.

Lewin, K. (1952) Group decision and social change, in *Readings in social psychology* (eds. G.E. Swanson, T.M. Newcomb & E.L. Hartley) Henry Holt, New York pp. 459–473.

Lewin, K. (1946) Action research and minority problems. *Journal of Social Issues*, **2**, 34–46.

Marika, R., Ngurrwutthun, D., and White, L. (1992). Always together, Yaka Gana: Participatory research at Yirrkala as part of the development of Yolngu education. *Convergence*, **25 (1)**, 23–39.

McCarthy, T. (1978) *The critical theory of Jurgen Habermas*, MIT Press, Cambridge, MA.

MacIntyre, A. (1981) *After virtue*, Duckworth, London.

MacKinnon, C.A. (1989) *Towards a feminist theory of the state*, Harvard University Press, Cambride MA.

McTaggart, R. (1988) Accountability, power and public knowledge. *Curriculum Concerns*, **5 (1)**, 21–25.

McTaggart, R. (1989a) *Institutional impediments to cross-cultural action research*. Paper presented to the Participatory Research Conference: A Celebration of People's Knowledge, Calgary, Alberta, Canada.

McTaggart, R. (1989b) *Principles for participatory action research*. Paper presented to The Third World Encounter on Participatory Research, Managua, Nicaragua.

McTaggart, R. (1989c) Bureaucratic rationality and the self-educating profession: The problem of teacher privatism, *Journal of Curriculum Studies*, **21 (4)**, 345–361.

McTaggart, R. (1989d) Reducing teachers to technicians: The role of the Biological Sciences Curriculum Study, *Australian Science Teachers Journal*, **35 (2)**, 35–43.

McTaggart, R. (1991a) Principles for participatory action research. *Adult Education Quarterly*, **41 (3)**, 168–187.

McTaggart, R. (1991b) Western institutional impediments to Aboriginal education. *Journal of Curriculum Studies*, **23 (4)**, 297–325.

McTaggart, R. (1991c) *Community movements and school reform: A new coalition for action research*. Keynote address to the Biennial Conference of the Australian Curriculum Studies Association, Adelaide, July.

McTaggart, R. (1992) Confronting accountability: Resisting transnational corporate ideology. *Curriculum Perspectives*, **12 (1)**, 72–78.

Merchant, C. (1980) *The death of nature: Women ecology and scientific revolution*, Harper and Row, New York.

Mernissi, F. (1987) *Beyond the veil: Male-female dynamics in modern Muslim society*, Indiana University Press, Bloomington IN.

Nandy, A. (1983) *The intimate enemy: loss and recovery of self under Colonialism*, Oxford University, Oxford.

Nielsen, K. (1983) Emancipatory social science and social critique, in *Ethics, the social sciences, and policy analysis* (eds. D. Callahan and B. Jennings), Plenum, New York pp. 113–157.

Pusey, M. (1991) *Economic rationalism in Canberra: A nation building state changes its mind*, Cambridge University Press, Cambridge.

Rothbard, M. (1988, Winter) Bankers conspire to dominate the world. *Money World*, 24–54.

Rowland, R. (1991) *Living laboratories: Women and the new reproductive technologies*, MacMillan, Melbourne.

Said, E.W. (1978) *Orientalism*, Pantheon, New York.

Shiva, V. (1989) *Staying alive: Women, ecology and development*, Zed, London.

Spivak, G.C. (1988) *In other worlds: Essays in cultural politics*, Routledge, London.

Starhawk (1987) *Truth or dare: Encounters with power, authority and mystery*, Harper, San Francisco.

Tandon, R. (1988) Social transformation and participatory research, *Convergence*, **21 (2/3)**, 5–14.

Tomlinson, B. (1991) Development in the 1990s: Critical reflections on Canada's economic relations with the Third World, in *Conflicts of interest: Canada and the Third World* (eds J. Swift and B. Tomlinson), Between the Lines, Toronto.

Trainer, T.E. (1985) *Abandon affluence!* Zed, London.

Trainer, T.E. (1989) *Developed to death: Rethinking Third World development*, Green, London.

Tsolidis, G. (1986) *Educating Voula*, Ministry of Education, Victoria.

Tungutalum, Wangintawujimawu (Wanginti) (1990) Tiwi Pedagogy: Ngini Nginingawula Ngawurranungurumagi, in *Aboriginal pedagogy: Aboriginal teachers speak out, Blekbala Wei, Deme Navin, Yolngu Rom, and Ngini Nginingawula Ngawurranungurumagi* (eds. R. Bunbury, W. Hastings,

J. Henry and R. McTaggart), Deakin University Press, Geelong, Australia.

Wa Thiong'o, Ngugi (1986) *Decolonizing the mind: The politics of language in African literature*, James Currey, London.

Waring, M.J. (1988) *Counting for nothing: What men value and what women are worth*, Allen and Unwin, Sydney.

Yunupingu, B.D. (1988) *Language and power: The Yolngu rise to power at Yirrkala Community School*. Paper presented at the UNESCO Conference on Teacher Education, Batchelor, Northern Territory.

CHAPTER 7

The historical sociology of healthcare

Evan Willis

INTRODUCTION

At its most basic, a research method is a means of 'knowing' about the social world. It represents one particular means of answering the fundamental question about the basis of knowledge of the social world. How can we 'know' about the social world? There are three main answers to this epistemological question. One can know about others by either observing and listening, by asking, or by reading their accounts (either contemporary or historical). In this chapter I both argue for the legitimacy and indeed importance of historical research in the domain of health research methods, and outline some of the practical lessons that emerge from such research that others seeking to embark along a similar methodological road might consider.

Methodologically, the focus is upon the use of historical method. This term means the use of historical materials to critically inform and develop an understanding of events in the past. More than that however, this chapter considers a particular approach to the use of historical materials in the form of what is usually called historical sociology. The methodological issues will be considered in the context of a study of the historical sociology of medical occupations and the evolution of the division of labour in health care which started out life as a doctoral dissertation and was eventually published in shortened form, first in 1983 and then in a second edition in 1989 as *Medical Dominance*.

All research starts out with a general sense of intellectual problem in the sense of a question for investigation. That question, at its most basic level, must strike the individual researcher as quite intriguing or curious. In the specific case of sociology this question

is a sociological problem. The sociological problem that I began with
in this study was 'how is the dominance of doctors within the health
system to be explained?' In virtually any health setting, a patient will
encounter a wide range of health workers who belong to a number
of different occupations; clerks, nurses, doctors, orderlies, cleaners
and so on. These occupations are socially organized into a complex
hierarchy especially in formal health care settings such as hospitals.
At the apex of this hierarchy stands the medical profession, dominating
the health workforce in all respects: politically, socially and financially.
Explaining this phenomenon, which I chose to call medical dominance,
constituted the sociological problem for the study. I studied two
historical 'moments'; the production (initial achievement) of medical
dominance, and its reproduction (defence). In the latter I considered
how the phenomenon of medical dominance had been defended by
analysing three modes of control over other health professions and
examining the historical process by which dominance was achieved:
subordination (midwifery); limitation (optometry); and exclusion
(chiropractic).

In one of those occurrences which the sociology of science literature
tells us is not uncommon, a similar sort of sociological problem
occurred to other researchers in other countries at much the same time.
Working entirely independently, the sense of problem which gave
rise to these studies arose out of the seminal work of the American
sociologist Eliot Freidson (1970a). The result was several publications
in different parts of the world, which, to a considerable extent, all
dealt with the same phenomenon. In the UK it was the work of Gerald
Larkin (1983), in the USA that of Paul Starr (1983), and in Canada
that of David Coburn *et al* (1983). They were studies in historical
sociology and in the historical sociology of medical occupations. They
were sociological in the sense of engaging sociological theories with
the use of historical data about how the division of labour in health
care had evolved. My own Australian work was part of this tradition,
the methodological issues associated with which are the focus of this
chapter.

The history of health and illness has been studied by researchers
from a variety of discipline backgrounds and perspectives. The purpose
has mostly been to illuminate the present with evidence from the past.
In framing and articulating the research problem for investigation it
was necessary first to develop a position in relation to the various
approaches or conceptual frameworks that existed. Three broad
traditions are identifiable: that of medical history, the social history
of medicine and the historical sociology of healthcare. Each has a
considerable heritage of research (though the first two more than the
third) and each had contributed much to our understanding of the
past in this area. In other words my aim in outlining these traditions

is not a territorial one. The process of embarking on research in general however involves locating the project within the existing literature. This requires developing a detailed understanding not only of existing empirical studies (one does not want to reinvent the wheel after all), but also of the sorts of conceptual and theoretical approaches that have informed previous work. In the next section I shall articulate this process of developing the theoretical framework with which *Medical Dominance* was written.

FROM MEDICAL HISTORY TO THE SOCIAL HISTORY OF MEDICINE

The original and still probably the most common approach to the history of health and illness has been termed 'medical history'. It is also the approach furthest from that taken in my study. While research from this perspective has contributed substantially to our understanding of the history of health care, in particular in the detail of its empirical investigation, its utility has been diminished by the approach taken. Usually conducted by medical practitioners with a historical bent, this approach has most often explicitly eschewed any concern with any of the underlying theoretical issues which are a crucial part of study in this field. The result is that the assumptions in relation to these theoretical issues remain implicit rather than explicitly addressed, revealed most clearly in the choice of research question. As Rosenberg (1971) argues:

> Most studies of the physician tend ... towards the episodic and anecdotal, emphasizing the atypical, even the quaint and quack at the expense of systematic consideration of patient care. The majority of institutional studies, moreover, tend to be construed in the narrowest of internal terms: histories of hospitals, of associations, of societies, based on one dimensional narrative of overt incident supplemented by arbitrary biographical compilation.

Although left implicit, such an approach takes definite positions in relation to the underlying theoretical and epistemological debates. These positions arise out of the contemporary medical world view based upon a particular paradigm of knowledge – that of western scientific medicine. Medical history often involves applying those assumptions backwards in time in order to trace how the state of knowledge we have today has been arrived at.

The purpose of this intellectual endeavour often appears to be legitimation of current medical practice. The course of medical history is often assumed from this perspective to be a process of linear development leading up to the present day; the past is combed for those elements of medical practice, which, from the perspective of present day medicine, have some validity. Ignored within this perspective are those developments which from the perspective of the present day constituted blind alleys and patently wrong turnings. More than that however, as Hicks (1982) argues, much of conventional medical history regards as unproblematic either the definition of the particular disease prevailing at the time or the understanding of the meaning of the disease. Such an approach derives from the paradigm of medical knowledge on which it is based with a positivistic methodological basis reflected in an emphasis on 'the facts'. By studying these apparently solid events of medical breakthroughs and discoveries, the belief is that the 'truth' of what actually occurred will be more and more achieved. The data is assumed to be self-evident, but as Figlio (1971) argues this assumption:

> ... automatically isolates the endeavour called 'scientific' or 'medical' advancement from its social context ... the solid record of the history of medicine, with its cautious abstinence from interpretation or evaluation is deceptive, because it reinforces in an implicit and unimpeachable way the currently held views of medicine and does this in the name of the 'historical perspective'.

The study of the history of healthcare, however, began to attract others to the field from the 1970s. These researchers were trained in disciplines other than medicine and levelled a powerful critique at the traditional medical history approach. In the process, the second approach emerged, that of the social history of healthcare. Whereas the medical history approach stressed the primacy of biological and scientistic processes over social and political ones, the social history approach emphasized the reverse (Rosenberg, 1970; McKeown, 1970; Grob, 1977; Woodward and Richards, 1977). This tradition of research differed from the former both empirically and methodologically.

Empirically, the need to locate an understanding of how healthcare and its treatment had evolved, not only from the perspective of present day knowledge but more importantly in the social context of the time, became the differentiating feature from conventional medical historical accounts. The sense of research problem for investigation then much more involved contextualizing what passed for medical treatment of the day, in terms of the social conditions which existed then, rather than only from the perspective of what turned out with the benefit of historical hindsight to be 'correct' today. There is thus a sense of openness about the manner in which these historical accounts are developed. Medical treatment did eventually go down this path of development, but at each stage there were other alternative paths along which it could and did develop. There is none of the sense of inevitability and linear development that has tended to characterize more conventional medical historical accounts. Rather the focus is upon political, social and economic processes that affected the manner in which health care was, and is, provided. The focus also reproduced the 'history from below' tendencies identified as characteristic of social history in general by Hobsbawm (1970). Medical history tended to present the medical view of the world to the exclusion of those of patients; the social history of healthcare by contrast considered the history of social relations between practitioners and their patients.

Methodologically, the social history of healthcare has also become gradually more differentiated from the medical history approach. As the specifically social history approach in general emerged, this approach began to be applied to the health area. A cautionary note apparent from a sense of perspective gained by being located outside the northern hemisphere is that in terms of their approaches to the study of social history, there exist differences in approach between different countries so that some cross-national variations are apparent which makes it hazardous to discuss 'the' social history approach. From the French Annales school, which for many originated the social history focus from the 1930s (e.g. Aries, 1960), to the development of social history in the UK and the USA (Calhoun, 1987), some differences are apparent which are beyond the scope of this chapter.

In general, a methodological difference is apparent in the way in which the data is approached and analysed. White (1990) summarizes this difference:

> ... historical data do not just exist 'out there' for us to go and find. We have to know what it is in the past that we are looking for – that is, what is relevant to us today – before we can find it. In other words ... history itself is constructed in the light of a given set of criteria and assumptions about what is relevant and who the significant set of actors were: and in full recognition that these criteria and assumptions are themselves the result of historical processes.

In other words, the degree to which the theoretical and epistemological underpinnings of a particular study within a particular approach to the history of healthcare, may be thought of as a continuum. The poles of this continuum are degrees of implicitness or explicitness of these underpinnings. At one pole then, is the medical history approach where the underpinnings are usually left entirely implicit, being of a taken-for-granted nature. Interpretation of the data is most often minimal and usually studiously avoided as if the 'facts speak for themselves'. The social history of healthcare approach is more towards the centre of this continuum, where the theoretical and epistemological underpinnings are beginning to be made more explicit. There is recognition methodologically that the 'facts' do not 'speak for themselves' but must be interpreted and placed within an explanatory framework in order to 'make sense'.

From social history to historical sociology of healthcare

The third approach to studying the history of healthcare is historical sociology. How exactly historical sociology differs in approach from the social history approach is again complicated somewhat by the different traditions in different parts of the world. In the British context, social history has traditionally been more closely identified with historical sociology; which is to say that much social history has been conducted with a clear sense of sociological problem. In other countries, such as the USA, where there has been a resurgence of interest in historical sociology recently, the two intellectual endeavours have tended to be more separate (Skocpol, 1984).

The argument here is that the continuum of implicitness/explicitness that was outlined above enables a distinction, albeit blurred, between social history and historical sociology. The latter is closest to the pole of explicitness in the sense of making clear the theoretical and epistemological foundations upon which the particular study rests. In terms of the British and American differences identified above, we can say that the tradition of British social history is closer to the pole of explicitness and therefore to historical sociology than the American tradition of social history has tended to be.

An explicit concern with the underlying theoretical traditions means of course, in this as in other fields of sociology, that there will be different approaches within historical sociology to studying the subject matter, even the same subject matter at times. In some senses therefore, it is appropriate to speak of historical sociologies reflecting a diversity of theoretical and resultant methodological approaches. Certainly historical sociology can be approached in either a qualitative or quantitative manner. On the theoretical side, in some cases, authors will explicitly identify the theoretical tradition within which they work. At other times there is enough conceptual discussion for the reader to be able to work it out for themselves. This is apparent in the series of studies that analysed the rise of the medical profession identified earlier. This of course allows the important sociological question to be posed (empirical differences aside) of which account provides the most sociologically useful or plausible analysis? So far, I have not seen this question precisely addressed. The pole of the continuum represented by historical sociology however is based upon the approach that '. . . doing history is an inherently political act in which data, concepts and explanations are "constructs" developed by and dependent upon the perspective of the researcher' (White, 1990). This hallmark, characteristic of sociological approaches, really reflects what is in effect one of the central insights of the sociology of science and knowledge, that technical knowledge can only be determined by taking account of the social context. In other words, that the claim to being 'the truth' can only be evaluated in the context of the social and political processes that produced it. The importance of Freidson's work lies in the application of this insight to the health arena as Hicks (1982) has argued.

The difference of historical sociology from both the other two approaches is reflected also in the choice of subject matter. The social history approach attempts to understand the health issues of the day in their social context as a means of illuminating present day issues. As McKeown (1970) argues it 'is essentially an operational approach which takes its terms of reference from difficulties confronting medicine in the present day'. He uses the example of hospital histories to illustrate:

> The task which remains for the social historian, is to interpret the evolution of hospitals against the background of the major problems which now confront them: provision of services of adequate standard for all classes of patient; rational accommodation to the uses and limitations of technology; reorientation of services of teaching centres; restriction of costs; extension of research into neglected areas, particularly in the applied field (McKeown, 1970).

The historical sociology approach, by contrast, more often takes its sense of problem to be a more strictly and therefore sometimes a more narrowly sociological one. Such a sociological problem may have policy implications of the sort that McKeown outlines, but that is not intrinsic to the enterprise in the way it tends to be for the social history approach. So, in *Medical Dominance* the sense of sociological problem for investigation is the relationship between technical and social factors in the evolution of the division of labour in healthcare to the point experienced today. In other words, it considers the relative importance of developments in science and technology, as against social and political processes considered more broadly in terms of the society as a whole.

But what makes it sociological? The defining feature of sociological research in particular, from my perspective, is using the theories of the discipline of sociology and the concepts that derive from them to analyse and 'make sense of' empirical data in order to illuminate and ultimately answer the sense of sociological problem posed for investigation in the first place. The theoretical traditions of the discipline are each based on a bedrock set of underlying epistemological assumptions about the social world and the relationship between the individual and society within it. Out of these traditions come a set of conceptual tools; individually and collectively useful for analysing and making sense of the empirical data being collected. Each conceptual tool is located however in a particular theoretical tradition. The process of what is called 'theorizing your concepts' in first developing the research and then subsequently writing that section of the overall report usually known as 'the literature review', involves locating each of the major conceptual tools used to make the analysis, in that theoretical tradition out of which it derives. Specifying the tools to be used for the analysis, then involves progressively narrowing down the available options, critiquing each in turn until the researcher specifies what will actually be used.

Having located *Medical Dominance* in the traditions of research on the history of healthcare, I will now consider several of the major methodological issues associated with the study in more detail. These are the relationship between theory and data, the question of evidence, especially the problem of contextual validity of the material being gathered, and the technical nature of the issues under consideration.

THE RELATIONSHIP BETWEEN THEORY AND EVIDENCE

The relationship between the unobservable (the conceptual/theoretical) and the observable (empirical evidence) may usefully be conceptualized by analogy as a house. According to this analogy, there are three parts which make up the building construction we call a house: the foundations, the framework and the covering (glass, wood, bricks). By analogy, the foundations may be thought of as the bedrock assumptions about major epistemological debates that underlie the social sciences, the framework as the theoretical component and the covering as the evidence of data that is used to cover the framework and provides the external appearance of the building. Non-observable concepts link and attach the theoretical framework to the data or evidence in the same way as the weatherboards or bricks are attached to the frame by nails or mortar.

All houses have foundations and a framework, otherwise there is no way of ordering and giving shape to the covering that is attached. The foundations will shape and give order to the framework to be attached to it in the same way as the underlying philosophical 'bedrock' assumptions will shape the framework built upon it. Yet sometimes the frame is not at all visible and can only be understood implicitly by the shape of the overall building. At other times the framework and foundations are much more apparent, perhaps, without stretching the analogy too much, like exposed beams. This is how the continuum of implicitness/explicitness outlined earlier can be located. The theoretical framework orders and gives form to the evidence. From the theoretical framework comes the research questions to be asked. These are then 'fleshed out' (to mix metaphors for a moment) by evidence using concepts. Without a conceptual and theoretical framework built upon philosophical foundations, the flesh can have no shape or order.

So, *Medical Dominance*, as an instance of historical research in the health field has these three components. It is based first upon foundations which are, broadly speaking, informed by the Marxist tradition of sociological thought. That tradition makes certain assumptions about the social world and how it operates. The assumption was made for instance, consistent with the position taken in what is known as the consensus/coercion debate, that coercion and conflict rather than consensus have been the means by which the division of labour in healthcare has evolved. The medical profession has not come to dominate the social structure of health care delivery because 'everybody agreed' that this was the most appropriate way to organize a health system, but as a consequence of the exercising of power and authority in which other health professions came to be controlled by medicine. All other health workers operate within relations of domination and subordination to the medical profession and experience different modes of domination as outlined above; either subordination, limitation or exclusion.

Arising from these foundations is the framework of the study. This is constructed from the existing literature as conceptual tools are developed to shape the emerging structure. The existing literature will be of a wide variety. In *Medical Dominance* it drew upon two whole areas: both the existing traditions of historical research in the health field (the history of medicine and the social history of healthcare), as well as the existing sociological literature. In this case, as with other researchers, the seminal work was that of Eliot Freidson (1970a) who analysed the social structure of healthcare in terms of the concept of 'professional dominance'. While acknowledging the significance of his work, two limitations are important. First, there was no detail on how the social structure of healthcare delivery got to be like that; that was not his intention after all, but it generated a research question that occurred to others in different parts of the world as well. The current structure of healthcare delivery is the current endpoint of a long historical process; tracing the evolution of the division of labour would therefore be interesting and relevant (and make a suitable PhD topic).

Secondly, though, the theoretical frame that Freidson used to construct his building, from the point of view of the foundations of my study was less useful. The conventional explanation for the dominance of the medical profession (particularly from members themselves and medical historians) has been and still is that its position is the result of developments in science and technology. According to this explanation, which I called 'technological determinist', the shape of the social structure of healthcare is the result of the developments in medical science and medical technologies, which have resulted in the profession that knows most about these things being in control. Freidson's explanation was a major advance on this explanation but looking out from my foundations did not go far enough. The study made the argument that, historically speaking, contrary to the accepted medical orthodoxy that developments in technology were responsible for creating (determining) the hierarchy of health workers, historical investigation showed the reverse. Hierarchy preceded technology, and developments in science and technology were used by the medical profession to strengthen their portion of dominance. The question to be explained then, was how did the hierarchy originate in the first place? To answer this question involved looking outside the health sector itself to the wider society, organized as it was along class lines resulting from a particular means of organizing economic life known as capitalism. For my study as for others (McKinlay, 1977), while Freidson showed the way conceptually speaking, his own analysis did not go far enough. For this reason, I used the term 'medical dominance' as an alternative to 'professional dominance' to differentiate it. In this way, constructing the frame involves 'theorizing your concepts', working out how they will be used in the study.

With the framework erected, the task of covering it with bricks or wood can proceed. The framework provides certain kinds of questions that will guide the empirical investigation. In my case, the framework gave rise to an interest in certain sorts of evidence. Here the 'medical history approach' was often useful in pointing in the direction of interesting historical leads to follow up. I was looking for influences, particularly business (corporate class) influences which shaped the division of labour. So in my case, this being obviously a relevant issue, I investigated as carefully as the available records would allow, the role of major philanthropic trusts, particularly international ones such as the Rockefeller and Carnegie foundations, in shaping the Australian healthcare system. I was also interested in the question of how developments in medical knowledge and technologies got taken up and used. Here questions of 'who by?' were relevant. An early example I uncovered was Sister Elizabeth Kenny, a remarkable nurse in the Australian state of Queensland in the 1930s who developed a means of treatment for poliomyelitis which was totally at odds with medical orthodoxy of the day. Conventional medical treatment involved immobilization of the affected limb whereas Kenny's method involved exercise. At first ridiculed and opposed by medicine, her method was gradually accepted and eventually adopted, becoming orthodox medicine with little acknowledgement of its origins as its success became increasingly apparent (Willis, 1979).

This position on the relationship between sociological theory and (historical) data is different, it should be noted, from that tradition known as 'grounded theory' (Glaser and Strauss, 1968). Indeed, there is apparent within sociology at present and within the sociology of health and illness in particular, something of a fashionable concern with this approach. Fuelled by the growth in popularity of qualitative methods, grounded theory has become the most common method by which these researchers, in either historical or contemporary contexts, seek to link the observable (data) with the unobservable (the conceptual/theoretical). In my view however, this approach to the relationship between theory and data (much of it carried out by postgraduate students) is based on a fairly simplistic notion of what it means to 'ground' your theory and indeed of what Glaser and Strauss themselves meant by the term. Social analysis can only be performed by exposing the data to the concepts with which it is being analysed. These concepts emerge, not in empiricist fashion out of the data itself but from the literature, both theoretical and from other substantive studies. Without a framework, after all, a building cannot have shape.

It should be said that a frequent objection to the approach that I have outlined as following in *Medical Dominance* is that specifying in advance your conceptual or theoretical framework will constrain, shape and determine your findings; that the structures will *a priori* determine the findings to be made in a particular field. Contrary to this, I would argue, via the house analogy, that the framework and the covering have to emerge together to give the overall building its shape. If the covering does not work out or will not fit (the so-called counter-factuals), or the end result does not meet the criteria of aesthetics or whatever, then the framework has to be amended. The grounded theory approach however often represents an attempt to construct a building by beginning with the covering and constructing the frame later. Clearly even a temporary frame is required to even begin to construct a house.

The approach followed in the study under consideration involved a continual 'dialogue' between the theory and the data. I went to 'the field' with a clear idea of what I was looking for, but on the basis of what was found there the theoretical frame required modification. With modification, the theoretical framework was more adequate but required still more modification and fine tuning. In this way the study as a whole emerged. Referring back to the framework was important in both in serving as a reminder of what questions had been started with and also in signposting where to go next in the search.

In other words while assuming the primacy of the object of study, 'facts' do not speak for themselves. Historical accounts are produced from negotiations between epistemological assumptions, theoretical concepts and methods, **and** from available evidence which has a demonstrable existence independent of the theory. The study is not just an illustration or refinement of the theory, but an attempt to understand and explain what occurred. Outlining concepts and defining terms is not specifying what is to be found in the historical materials, nor does it provide a basis for discounting disconfirmatory evidence, but instead outlines the foundations and frame on which the historiographic analysis can be constructed.

THE PROBLEM OF EVIDENCE

The other methodological issue to be considered is the question of what constitutes evidence in this field. The usual limitations of historiographic data considering validity and reliability are apparent in historical sociology as well. The most interesting aspects of a phenomenon, from the point of view of the study in hand, may never be written down, the records may be lost or destroyed. The available evidence is often difficult to access and may be guarded by a protective gatekeeper wary of exposing the past deeds of individuals or organizations to the sort of critical analysis that social science research usually involves. As an accurate picture of what took place the available evidence is only rarely adequate to generate a complete account of what occurred. There are bound to be huge gaps in the available evidence. In my view you have to be open about these and constantly guard against the temptation to claim more than the data allows. At the same time, pursuing the general methodological criterion of reliability, it is important to make very clear the sources on which your argument is based, so that others are able to check the basis for your argument and potentially argue against your interpretation. How can the criteria of validity be pursued?

There are a number of responses. First, the aim, as with all historical research, is for what Deising (1971) calls 'contextual validity'; that is assessing each piece of evidence in the context of other pieces of evidence. This was particularly an issue given the amount of rhetoric that has flowed in the political processes under investigation. Corroboration was sought, not only from historical documents, legislation, journals and other historical sources of a written nature, but also by interviewing or doing 'oral histories' of what Gorden (1975) calls 'special respondents'. Conventional historical research often prefers to deal only with those events where the participants have long since passed away. In this case however respondents were selected because their social or occupational position enabled them to give information directly relevant to the study's objectives.

Approximately 30 interviews were conducted with respondents who had been directly involved in the production and reproduction of medical dominance, being careful, wherever possible, to interview respondents on both 'sides' of the political debates under investigation.

Assessing the contextual validity of evidence then could be pursued in three different ways: comparing evidence given in one document with that given in another; comparing documentary accounts with verbal accounts of events given in interviews; and comparing interview with interview.

Conventional historiography also has a distinct preference for primary sources because of the difficulties of interpretation. In this case however, given the broad scope of the study, while some of the historical research was original, much of it involved secondary analysis of existing sources. In doing so, as much of the original sources as could be checked, were. In some cases with some narrowly situated studies, data collected for a different purpose was recast and used in this study.

The technical arguments

This is another issue concerning the interpretation of the data. At times, the issues under consideration were highly technical ones, as they often are in health research. For the social scientist interested in such issues, understanding the technical debates is therefore an issue. Indeed, conventional medical historians have been known to argue that holding a medical degree is an essential prerequisite to adequate research in this field (see Hicks, 1982).

Differences over therapy however become differences between therapists and the organizations that represent them. The evidence then becomes the nontechnical data concerning the evolution of the medical profession and other healthcare professions. At the same time though, the technical issues can never be entirely separated from the nontechnical issues. Cognizant of this, and aware that nothing will destroy the credibility of a social science researcher in the health field faster in general than 'getting it very wrong' on some relatively straightforward issue, in this study (as in all subsequent research), at some point before publication I have the manuscript read by someone with medical training who is able to comment with this concern specifically in mind. In the case of this study, I was fortunate to have an associate supervisor who was medically qualified.

CONCLUSION

The historical method is an underutilized but legitimate and important methodological approach in health research particularly when it entails more than just content analysis of documents from the past. The historical sociological approach has much to contribute to an understanding both of sociological problems in general and to health policy questions in particular. Its contribution lies in elucidating the 'lessons from the past' which are many in healthcare. A sense of historical perspective is important so often to balance the historical nature of much contemporary research and writing on healthcare. So many of the major health issues of our time, on which a considerable amount of research effort is expended, have an important historical dimension that is often overlooked, cursorily treated, or ignored. Historical sociology, in any of its theoretical guises, represents an approach and a method that is capable of making a contribution to health research as significant as any other social science methodologies.

REFERENCES

Aries, P. (1960) *Centuries of Childhood* Penguin, Harmondworth.

Calhoun, C. (1987) History and sociology in Britain: a review article. *Comparative Studies in Society and History*, **29** (3), pp. 615–25.

Coburn, D., Torrance, G. and Kaufert, J. (1983) Medical dominance in Canada in historical perspective: the rise and fall of medicine? *International Journal of Health Services*, **13** (3), pp. 407–32.

Deising, P. (1971) *Patterns of Discovery in the Social Sciences*, Aldine, Chicago.

Figlio, K. (1971) The historiography of scientific medicine: an invitation to the human sciences. *Comparative Studies in Society and History*, **19** (3), pp. 262–86.

Freidson, E. (1970a) *Professional Dominance: The Social Structure of Medical Care*, Aldine, Chicago.

Freidson, E. (1970b) *Profession of Medicine*, Dodd Mead, New York.

Glaser, B. and Strauss, A. (1968) *The Discovery of Grounded Theory*, Aldine, Chicago.

Grob, G. (1970) The social history of medicine and disease in America: problems and possibilities. *Journal of Social History*, **10** (4), pp. 391–409.

Gorden, R. (1975) *Interviewing Strategy: Techniques and Tactics*, Dorsey, Homewood, III.

Hicks, N. (1982) Medical history and the history of medicine in *New History: Studying Australia Today* (eds W. Mandle and G. Osborne), Allen and Unwin, Sydney, pp. 69–81.

Hobsbawm, E. (1970) From social history to the history of society, *Daedalus*, **100**, pp. 20–39.

Larkin, G. (1983) *Occupational Monopoly and Modern Medicine*, Tavistock, London.

McKeown, T. (1970) A sociological approach to the history of medicine. *Medical History* **14**, pp. 342–51.

McKinlay, J.B. (1977) The business of good doctoring or doctoring as good business: reflections on Freidson's view of the medical game. *International Journal of Health Services*, 7, 3, pp. 459–88.

Rosenberg, C. (1970) The medical profession, medical practice and the history of medicine in *Modern Methods in the History of Medicine*, E. Clarke, Althone Press, London, pp. 22–35.

Skocpol, T. (1984) *Vision and Method in Historical Sociology*, Cambridge University Press, New York.

Starr, P. (1983) *The Social Transformation of American Medicine*, Basic Books, New York.

White, K. (1990) Towards a social history of the hospital, in *Medicine and Society* (eds D. Turnbull, B. Butcher, L. Farrell, S. Jacobs and J. McCulloch), Deakin University, Geelong, pp. 1–13.

Willis, E. (1979) Sister Elizabeth Kenny and the evolution of the occupational division of labour in health care, *Australian and New Zealand Journal of Sociology*, 15, 3, pp. 30–9.

Willis, E. (1989) *Medical Dominance*, (rev. edn), Allen & Unwin, Sydney.

Woodward, J. and Richards, D. (eds) (1977) *Health Care and Popular Medicine in Nineteenth Century England: Essays in the Social History of Medicine*, Croom Helm, London.

CHAPTER 8

Phenomenological method in nursing: theory vs. reality

Bev Taylor

INTRODUCTION

Since my earliest recollections of relatively mature reflective thought, I have been a person who has believed firmly in the benefits of making a strategic plan for important events in my life. Projections of likely situations and ways of approaching them have been my salvation in the immediacy of 'life's little trials', so in my postgraduate student life the academic requirement to produce a research proposal outlining a method, prior to embarking on an area of study, seemed a reasonable thing to do. What I failed to recognize on the research occasion I will describe now and in many other less formal personal occasions in which I have formulated plans of action, was that although at the time it seemed the best possible avenue, I was under no obligation to remain wedded permanently to that plan.

The title of this chapter comes from the realization of a lesson I am constantly learning in my professional and personal life: things change and courses of possible action change with them. Recognizing the differences between theories of ideal conditions and realities of transpiring circumstances, is an on-going lesson. This chapter recounts my PhD research experience and suggests that the terrain between the theory of idealized intentions and the reality of contextualized action can be traversed using a cognitive map, which allows for detours according to changing research conditions and expectations.

THE 'THEORY' OF MY INTENTIONS

Originally there were few things about which I was clear in relation to the research. I knew I wanted to research the nurse–patient relationship in a clinical setting and that I wanted to look especially at a phenomenon I had noticed in my own practice (Taylor, 1988), which had been dubbed by Professor Alan Pearson (1988) as 'ordinariness in nursing', but beyond that, anything seemed possible. Being a novice researcher, initially I relied heavily on the guidance of my research supervisors in matters of methodology and method.

A research journal I kept of my experiences records a process that began with wide parameters of grandiose ideas, and focused down gradually to a manageable PhD project. Through a series of exploratory and evaluative activities, I was projected forwards towards the goal of a PhD award, mobilized by a combination of sensitive research supervision and my own determined pragmatic mentality. It is not my intention to describe every twist and turn in that pathway, suffice to say that I began as a tentative researcher, barely able to toddle along conceptually, and gradually I became surer and safer on my feet. The assistance of my supervisors and a growing confidence in my own ability to be attentive to the features of the research context assisted my progress. Eventually I was able to develop and defend the use of a research method, which reflected the contextual features of the research setting as well as some assumptions of an underlying methodology.

Initial plans and feelings

The decision to centre my research in a phenomenological perspective did not come automatically. I spent a period of clarifying my research interest, trying to become clearer about what it was I wanted to know about ordinariness in nursing. Initially, I imagined that I might work in a birthing unit with midwives and explore ordinariness through facilitating natural birth processes. A preliminary tour of the unit, which was still under construction at that time, revealed a doctor-dominated structure of obstetric practice masquerading as midwifery, in a system set up with interventionary equipment stored behind the veneer of a 'normalized' bedroom setting and with an organizational policy that midwives would be obliged to act as assistants only in a private hospital system, which neither recognized nor valued the autonomy of their birthing skills and knowledge. Under these conditions, in my mind, ordinariness in nursing became linked to questions of empowerment of mothers and midwives and the spectre of using a critical methodology to lead a bloody revolution against seemingly unassailable odds seemed too great a challenge for me at that stage of my research career.

I knew I wanted to be reasonably comfortable with my research interest for the time our 'courtship' needed to last, so my retreat

from the 'revolution' was mainly on selfish grounds, knowing that
that specific interest could be taken up later as postdoctoral research,
when I was an older and wiser person. This change of heart, however,
led me to realize that what I really wanted to know about was the
phenomenon of ordinariness in nursing itself. Realizing that I wanted
to explore the nature of this thing called ordinariness, I moved to a
methodology which for me dealt with the assumptions of getting to
know more about a particular phenomenon of interest, that is,
phenomenology.

My preconceptions of phenomenology were different from my
experience of reading and thinking about it. I imagined that
phenomenology would be a fairly limited perspective with a readily
digestible literature of theoretical development. My naivety was
shattered into stunned awe by the writings of Spiegelberg (1976) who
used an historical perspective to describe the various forms of
phenomenology and by Heidegger (1962), who seemed to speak in
circular riddles as he explicated the nature of being and time. In
going on a journey into the arena of phenomenology, I realized that
my erroneous preconceptions were like trying to judge the distance
on a map without a clue to its scale, in the sense that 2 cm on a map
might equal 1 million km in real terms. I had not figured upon the
breadth and depth of one philosopher alone, let alone the works of
many and the subtle methodological connections between them.

With further reading, the stunned awe turned to absolute and high
pitched nervous anxiety, as the reality dawned on me that I had neither
the time nor the interest to pursue phenomenology *per se* in depth
and breadth. One of my supervisors caught the sense of my despera-
tion and reminded me that I was doing a PhD with a nursing focus;
the intention was not to be a philosopher, the intention was to use
phenomenology as a methodology from which to extract a method
for pursuing a nursing question. It was a matter of deciding on a form
of phenomenology that suited my research requirements and of
treating the remainder of phenomenology much as a traveller would,
who glances out of a window of a speeding train as it traverses a wide
and seemingly endless terrain. I realized that the particular form of
phenomenology I chose was to be a vehicle for mobilizing my thinking in relation to the research interest and that the matching method
would be the engine energizing that mobility.

My expectations about the research setting were informed to some
degree by working in the nursing unit during faculty practice time.
Under this arrangement, I was paid by the university and approved
by the hospital, to work as an honorary nurse practitioner for at least
20% of my academic time in a clinical setting, as a means of bridg-
ing the theory/practice gap in nursing and making my teaching of
nursing authentic to the students of nursing and to myself. I had

come to know some of the nurses and patients in the nursing unit and I was assured of their co-operation in my forthcoming research project. What I did not know was just what I would need to do to ensure that the nature of the phenomenon I was hoping to illuminate would 'come to light'.

THE REALITY OF MY EXPERIENCES

After much deliberation, I convinced my MPhil/PhD Defence Committee of the value of using a phenomenological method to bring out the meaning of the concept as perceived by the research participants (Langveld, 1978). The method involved a series of transformations through which the participants' impressions were to be processed to make the meaning clear, necessitating repeated and systematic analyses of the data with the people involved. Set out as 'theory' on paper, the method seemed ideal for the purposes of the study, however, the experience of putting the plan into action revealed context–dependent problems, which made the method unworkable in its original form.

Before the actual data collection began and after a 3-month delay waiting for the approval of a medically dominated hospital ethics committee, which had minimal idea of qualitative research methods, let alone methodologies such as phenomenology, I tried out the method with four patients in the nursing unit. I had been advised in a discussion with a visiting Professor of Nursing that a beneficial way of eliciting phenomenological accounts from participants was to have them describe a recent event in terms of the who, where, when, with whom of the situation, and as they speak, to have them enlarge on their accounts by seeking effective responses, through questions such as: 'How did you feel?', 'What were you thinking at the time?' This seemed easy enough, especially as I felt I knew each patient fairly well having been part of their intimate nursing care on several occasions before each interview.

I began by asking each patient to think of a recent interaction with a nurse. I then asked each patient to describe that situation and attempted to elicit their effective responses as I had been advised. I found that the patients did not elaborate fully on single encounters with nurses, rather they tended to refer briefly to a variety of situations. My attempts to bring patients back to a particular event became directive to the point that I doubted that the participants were really describing the meaning in the experience for themselves, rather they seemed to be accommodating my need to be true to my interviewing method.

Processing the participants' responses also proved to be difficult. The transformation process required repeated discussions with the participants, so that the researcher's and each participant's impressions could be counter-checked. The reality dawned on me rapidly that if I were to use this transformation process I would need to set up and keep multiple engagements with each participant – with their changing fortunes of health and illness and my own meagre research funds, the method would become unworkable. Added to this, the patients' tendencies to recall wide-ranging recollections of a mosaic of experiences with nurses meant that elaborations on specific nursing behaviours would be difficult to assess.

In short, as I tried it and considered it more and more, I liked this particular method less and less. This situation created a fair amount of concern, given that I had put the plan out for public scrutiny to my supervisors, the defence committee, peers, and university and hospital ethics committees, and they, with varying degrees of acceptance, seemed to think it was OK. At a very basic level I thought to myself: 'It must be OK if everyone likes it'. In my research journal I recorded feelings of ambivalence in the form of questions, such as: 'What is required for a PhD?', 'To what extent am I bound by my "word" to the defence committee and others about my anticipated research method?'

Alice in the wonderland of phenomenology

Having invested myself in the research process, things seemed to happen all at once and in all directions, leaving me somewhat bemused as I made my way through it all. At the time that I was to begin the data collection in earnest, I was reading and thinking about phenomenology and discovering that the differences between certain philosophers were indeed profound. I realized that Husserl's commitment to the idea of transcendental phenomenology (Husserl, 1960, 1964, 1970, 1980) came from his search for a science of essences, an 'apodictic beginning point, for an indubitable epistemic foundation', which in itself discovers 'Being' (Stapleton, 1983). For Husserl, transcendental consciousness was that sense of being that could be experienced by going beyond the realms of people and things to find the essence of a phenomenon itself.

The phenomenological method suggested by Husserl required that one suspend unquestioning acceptance of the prephilosophical or natural attitude of taken-for-grantedness, which is situated in a web of relationships to things and people in the natural world, to take on the philosophical attitude, which demands to know the reasons why things are as they are. The transition from the prephilosophical to the philosophical attitude was through phenomenological reduction or 'bracketing', which narrowed one's attention in such a way as to be able to discover rational principles underlying the phenomenon of concern.

Husserl claimed that there was a residue, which remained after bracketing; that something which remained was the ego itself. In order to escape the subject–object dualism of Cartesian thought and subsequent philosophy, Husserl referred to this ego as 'transcendental consciousness', because it embraced both subjective and objective elements. He contended that ego could not be conceived apart from conscious life, thus consciousness was always intended towards ego. The phenomenological epoche (reduction, bracketing) was therefore a means by which the natural world could be reduced to a transcendental consciousness or transcendental subjectivity, through which 'consciousness was purified and only phenomena remained. Analysing the phenomena, in turn, revealed the basic structure of consciousness itself' (Husserl, 1980).

I began to understand something of Husserl's view of phenomenology and found that it differed from Heidegger's. Husserl was Heidegger's teacher and colleague and authors (Kockelmans, 1967; Spiegelberg, 1970, 1976; Stapleton, 1983; Sukale, 1976) have elaborated on their personal and philosophical differences. Sukale (1976) concluded that 'the basic difference between Husserl and Heidegger boiled down to their different interpretation of the concept of "world".' It was as though there were different two levels: the level of the natural world and the level below the natural world, from which all things sprang. Husserl was intent on reaching the world below, whilst Heidegger was concerned with Being-in-the-world, therefore, instead of trying to lay presuppositions to one side, Heidegger explored them as legitimate parts of Being.

Heidegger's main departures from Husserlian phenomenology were found in his book *Being and Time*. Heidegger (1962) began his book with a question about Being, placing his search firmly in the perspective of hermeneutical enquiry, that is, into the analysis and interpretation of language and text. Heidegger sought to establish the basis of philosophy as an historical analysis of existence, raising questions about Being and hermeneutical enquiry. Thus, Heidegger saw the task of philosophers as ontologists, seeking to unravel 'the universal structures of Being as they manifested themselves in the phenomena'. In using hermeneutical enquiry to pursue the question of Being, Heidegger effectively demonstrated the nature of 'Dasein', that is, the nature of human entities, who have some awareness of how to ask questions about Being, in as much as their Being-in-the-world as humans gives them some clues to the existence and nature of Being.

I discovered through reading that Heidegger's ontological use of the hermeneutic circle, transformed the scope, meaning and significance of it as described by Scheiermacher (1977) and Dilthey (1976), by moving hermeneutics away from its sole focus on texts, to interpret the human being through the understanding of Being implicit in Dasein. Dasein is the 'There-being' of people and things and the ways in which people can ask questions about Being, by virtue of living in a world of other people and things. Heidegger (1962) extended the hermeneutic circle to the ontological expression of Dasein, so that a fundamental ontology could be developed by an hermeneutic interplay between entities (expressions of Being) and sense (concern about Being).

For Heidegger, the hermeneutic circle aided in the interpretation of 'Dasein' itself as an understanding, caring mode of Being. 'Dasein' tied to the world the one who questioned, a place from whence no conscious separation was possible, given the nature of Being-in-the-world. For Husserl the ultimate intentional connection between the act of knowing and the thing as known, abided in 'pure consciousness' or in transcendence of the natural attitude, whereas, for Heidegger, it was in the whole of people's precognitive awareness, by virtue of their prior understanding of Being, by being inextricably immersed within it.

In naming Heidegger's particular brand of phenomenology, I realized that Heidegger's ontological phenomenology was concerned with existence, specifically human existence, or 'Dasein', so in that sense it was existential. However, the point of departure with his approach as existential phenomenology as such, was in his emphasis on an hermeneutic, which analysed the historically-situated self as a Being-in-the-world, thus it became an existential–ontological hermeneutic. For Heidegger, people were always arriving out of their past, deciding on their present and anticipating their future, the ultimate reality of which is death, thus the seeds to understanding Being itself and its phenomena, were in the historicity and temporality of people's Being-in-the-world.

On climbing out of the rabbit hole ...

After a period of meandering in the labyrinth of the literature, it was time to make a decision to surface with a firm decision about method. Whereas all of this reading and thinking was enjoyable, it also proved challenging, if somewhat frustrating. The method of transformation of interpretations that I had intended initially to use in my PhD research was essentially Husserlian in nature, therefore, this method raised some questions in my mind about Husserl's search for essences and transcendental consciousness. In the face of my new understandings, the tension in choosing this method was in the use of the terminology 'ground structure', which seemed to suggest certain universal principles reminiscent of positivistic understandings, which was an apparent contradiction for a methodology, that was seated in the moment of an experience and was concerned with on-going dialogue. I realized that if I doubted that the essence of things could be found by bracketing the world, the legitimacy of this method was doubtful for describing being within the experiences of the patients, the nurses and myself, as we interacted together in the world of the nursing unit.

Many published nursing research reports and journal articles to date have adopted an Husserlian view of phenomenology and therefore suggest some form of bracketing (Oiler, 1982, 1986; Omery, 1983; Parse, 1985, 1987, 1990; Reiman, 1986). A review of the literature revealed an uncritical acceptance of an Husserlian 'brand' of phenomenology as though it were the only type, with the exceptions of work of nursing scholars such as Paterson and Zderad (1976) who used existentialist perspectives, and Benner (1984), whose work was based mainly on Heideggerian assumptions.

I had been searching for a 'ready-made' phenomenological method such as the Van Kaam method (1959a,b), the Giorgi method (1975) or the Colaizzi method (1978) and I had not been able to locate one to meet the needs of the unique research contextual features and my needs as a person, nurse and researcher. The botttom line was that I could not in all fairness purport to be able to bracket my presuppositions about nursing, given my own experience of all the things that comprise my world, so I decided that I would have to discard the transformation method for the sake of methodological and personal congruency.

RECONCILING IDEALIZED INTENTIONS WITH THE REALITIES OF EXPERIENCE

Like Alice travelling through Wonderland, I was lost in the literature which became 'curioser and curioser', but my directions were clarified by people and insights along the way. Frequent dialogue with my research supervisors, discussions with friends, research peers and experts, led to the development of some inner stability about reasonable parameters of the research. I had already decided that the research aims were nursing related first and foremost, and that these were to be illuminated by a phenomenological perspective. Further reading led me to Gadamer and a compromise position to help sort out my cognitive dissonance about matching methodology to method.

Gadamer's major work, *Truth and Method* (1975) addressed the task of hermeneutics to explore philosophically the conditions of all understanding. Attempting to find out what the human sciences really were, that is, 'what kind of insight and what kind of truth' could be found in the human sciences, he set up a conflict between truth and method, which needed to address the question that if human sciences went beyond method and still had truth, then was truth itself beyond the question of method.

By exploring basic humanistic concepts and making an analysis of the experience of art, he sought to discover how understanding was possible. Gadamer (1975) decided that all understanding is hermeneutical, because hermeneutics is the 'basic being-in motion of there-being, which constitutes its finiteness and historicity and hence includes the whole experience of the world'. For Gadamer, the study of hermeneutics was ontological, being ultimately connected to the study of language, wherein Being could be understood. He resolved that the nature of the human sciences was in appreciating that all understanding is linguistic and can be thus examined through language.

Like Heidegger before him, Gadamer was convinced that understanding was not an epistemological problem, but that rather it was an ontological one. In avoiding Heidegger's tendency towards ontological absolutism, which was Heidegger's tendency to perceive all questions about knowing framed as enquiries about Being, Gadamer discussed ontology in terms of the linguisticity (language-based awareness) of all understanding and historicity (awareness of history).

Gadamer adopted Heidegger's view of the hermeneutic circle, that it was necessary in the ontology of understanding as an 'interplay of the movement of tradition' and its consequences (Gadamer, 1975). He determined that the tendency of the Enlightenment to attempt to eradicate prejudice was prejudicial in itself and that truth could be pursued by identifying the connections between truth and prejudice. He contended that it was the task of hermeneutics to make distinctions between true and false prejudices, by a process of effective historical consciousness. Gadamer suggested that effective historical consciousness was analogous to the I–Thou relationship (1975) in which openness to the other and willingness to be modified, created a dialogical relationship, that is, a mutual sharing of awarenesses.

Using the concept of horizon described by Husserl as the 'range of vision that includes everything that can be seen from a particular vantage point', Gadamer (1975) determined that a 'fusing of horizons' occurs in effective historical consciousness. The sum total of one's own horizon or ideas about a phenomenon is understood in order to understand another's and the conscious act of fusion of the two horizons is through an act of understanding, as the task of effective historical consciousness. Notions of effective historical consciousness and dialogical relationships resonated with my imaginings of how the research method might be informed.

At that point of my methodological search it seemed that, unlike the amorphous nature of Heidegger's unending abstractions, Gadamer provided practical suggestions for a phenomenological method. Gadamer (1975) used conversation as an example of the fusion of horizons, by noting that the merging of meaning that goes on is an instance of the linguisticality of understanding, as the 'concretation' of effective historical consciousness. The correctness of interpretation is decided by examining the degree of 'conformity to the horizon from which the interpretation is made and the prejudices that constitute the horizon (Hekman, 1986). Like Heidegger before him, Gadamer acknowledged the nature of human existence situated in the world of people and things and worked with those preconceptions as preunderstandings of Being.

These methodological assumptions legitimated a method which attested to people's particular experiences of Being-in-the-world. The method I compiled made no attempts to bracket presuppositions to find the essences of things, rather it acknowledged the importance of people's lived experiences by exploring the participants' worlds and the intersubjective meanings they found within them.

A method to fit the reality of the research context

In seeking to explicate the nature and effects of the phenomenon of ordinariness in nursing and to find whether or not the phenomenon enhanced the nursing encounter, I worked as a participant observer with six registered nurses in a Professorial Nursing Unit (PNU) in Australia. I was known to the nurses, because I had spent each Friday of the previous year working in the PNU as an Honorary Nurse Practitioner during my Faculty Practice in university-supported clinical time.

Having secured the necessary consent from all the people involved, I was present at each nurse–patient interaction, helping the respective nurses where appropriate with nursing care, such as attending to hygiene needs, dressing and elimination procedures and bed-making. The nurse–patient interactions were part of the usual nursing care acivities and each nurse interacted with four patients. My presence during the interaction was to give each of the participants a common ground for discussing their impressions of a recent nurse–patient interaction and as a background for discussing any other concerns they chose to raise in the course of our conversation.

Following each interaction, I wrote my impressions in a personal–professional journal and audiotaped conversations with the respective patients and nurses to gain their impressions. A pattern of order emerged quite naturally. I wrote my accounts during a resting phase for patients, following their nursing care activities. The nurses were always available to take time out from their clinical responsibilities later in the day, when the change of shift nurses came on duty, so the order of relating and recording impressions each time evolved quite effortlessly in the order of researcher, patient and nurse.

Following the phase of gathering of impressions from the nurse–patient interactions, I withdrew from the PNU to begin the phase of analysis and interpretation of the recorded impressions. I had some sense of what 'the thing' ordinariness in nursing might be; however, I was prepared to accept Gadamer's suggestion to approach the exploration of the phenomenon with open-mindedness and a willingness to be surprised and informed by what emerged.

Using a theoretical framework of the phenomenological concepts of lived experience, Dasein, Being-in-the-world and fusion of horizons as an underpinning methodology, an initial hermeneutical analysis and interpretation of the impressions generated qualities and activities indicative of the aspects of the phenomenon of ordinariness in nursing.

The qualities and activities were derived from an analysis of the transcribed interviews and my notes. Initially I read and re-read the text of each interaction, always keeping the contextual features of each interaction intact. Following this, a computerized word search package was used, which allowed me to thoroughly scan each interaction and extract text tagged to the specific contextual features of the participants' interactions.

Many qualities and activities emerged within each interaction, which included such things as: appreciating skilful nursing care; appreciating help; facilitating independence; facilitating learning; facilitating coping; facilitating comfort; facilitating acceptance of body image changes; facilitating changes; calming fears; building trust; giving confidence; allowing the experience to unfold; straight talking; tolerating one another's humanness and many more.

The qualities and activities related to the nurses' and patients' experiences as they were perceived by them and conveyed to me through their own unique use of language. After a period of immersion in the text of the transcribed interviews and a process of fusion with the text and my own impressions as part of my Being-in-the-world of the PNU, I categorized the respective qualities and activities into eight main parts. I gave the term 'aspects' to these groupings to denote their identities as parts of the phenomenon itself. The aspects of the phenomenon were named facilitation, fair play, familiarity, family, favouring, feelings, fun and friendship. No one aspect was seen as being greater or lesser than the others, they were simply grouped alphabetically for ease of reference.

The method I have described evolved out of the unique contextual features of the research and seemed to be methodologically congruent and effective. The unique contextual features of the research included those people and things that made it unique, for instance, those six nurses, 24 patients, and myself as participant/observer, who interacted in a particular place in a particular time to generate our own context specific understandings of the phenomenon under study. The method was based on certain methodological assumptions which resonated with my own experience and in as much as those assumptions can be reasoned to have sufficient epistemological veracity, they have formed the underpinning of a method which has the potential for describing the phenomenon of interest.

Lessons learned from the experience

The search for a method which fitted the requirements of the research was at times tortuous and disheartening, but never boring. I began the research process with certain preconceptions of what I might discover and found that the theory of my expectations was not in line with the reality of my experience. With the benefit of hindsight, I can now offer the following suggestions.

One of the first things to note is: 'It's OK!' and I do not mean this in a classic Australian 'She'll be right!' sense. Nothing is set in cement until the report or the thesis is submitted for appraisal. It is OK to change your mind about the method. It is OK to bleat about your insecurities as you move through periods of methodological uncertainty. It is OK to keep on discussing and clarifying your issues with others whose opinions you respect. It is OK to feel proud of your increasing understanding.

The following things worked for me and you may find them helpful in some ways for you. First, choose a research question or area you like and match it to a methdology you can tolerate for a protracted time; select supervisors you like as people and respect as experts and keep open communication channels with them. Be clear about the methodological assumptions underlying the method and decide whether methodological congruence is an issue for you.

CONCLUSION

The danger in giving advice is that it often sounds trite in as much as it reeks of so called common sense and seems too plain to be useful. Through the metaphor of a journey this chapter described my movement from the theory of a proposed method to the reality of an evolved method. The researcher who searches for and discovers a research method is similar to a traveller who sets out on a journey with an anticipated itinerary; sometimes things go to plan and sometimes things change according to contingencies along the way. I hope that the description of my travelling to find a methodologically congruent method helps you in some way with your anticipated research journey.

Benner, P. (1984) *From Novice to Expert: Uncovering the Knowledge Embedded in Clinical Practice*, Addison-Wesley, California.
Colaizzi, P. (1978) Psychological research as the phenomenologist views it, in *Existential Phenomenological Alternatives for Psychology* (eds R.S. Valle and M. King), Oxford University Press, New York, pp. 48–71.
Dilthey, W. (1976 trans.) in *Dilthey: Selected Writings* (ed. H.P. Rickman) Cambridge University Press, Cambridge.
Gadamer, H-G. (1975) *Truth and Method* (ed. and trans. G. Barden and J. Cumming), Seabury, New York.
Giorgi, A., Fischer, C.L. and Murray, E.L. (1975) *Duquesne Studies in Phenomenological Psychology*, Vol. 2., Duquesne University Press, Pittsburgh.
Heidegger, M. (1962) *Being and time* (trans. J. Macquarrie and E. Robinson). Harper and Row, New York.
Hekman, S.J. (1986) *Hermeneutics and the Sociology of Knowledge*, Polity Press, Cambridge.
Husserl, E. (1960) *Cartesian Meditations: An Introduction to Phenomenology*, (trans D. Cairns), Martinus Nijhoff, The Hague.
Husserl, E. (1964) *The Idea of Phenomenology* (trans. W.P. Alston and G. Nakhnikian), Martinus Nijhoff, The Hague.
Husserl, E. (1970) *The Crisis of the European Sciences and Transcendental Phenomenology*, Northwestern University Press, Evanston, Ill.
Husserl, E. (1980) *Phenomenology and the Foundations of the Sciences*, (trans. T.E. Klein and W.E. Pohl), Martinus Nijhoff, The Hague.
Kockelmans, J.J. (1967) (ed) *Phenomenology: The Philosophy of Edmund Husserl and its Interpretation*, Anchor Books, Doubleday and Company, Inc., Garden City, New York.
Langveld, M.J. (1978) The stillness of the secret place. *Phenomenology and Pedagogy*, 1 (1), pp. 181–9.
Oiler, C. (1982) The phenomenological approach in nursing research. *Nursing Research*, 31 (3), pp. 171–81.
Oiler, C. (1986) Phenomenology: the method, in *Nursing Research: A Qualitative Perspective* (eds. P. Munhall and C.J. Oiler), Appleton-Century-Crofts, Norwalk.
Omery, A. (1983) Phenomenology: A method for nursing research, *Advances in Nursing Science*, 5 (2), pp. 49–63.
Parse, R.R. (1985) *Nursing Research: Qualitative Methods*, Brady, Bowie.
Parse, R.R. (1987) *Nursing Science: Major Paradigms, Theories and Critiques*, W.B. Saunders, Philadelphia.
Parse, R.R. (1990) Parse's research methodology with an illustration of the lived experience of hope, *Nursing Science Quarterly*, pp. 9–17.
Paterson, J. and Zderad, L. (1976) *Humanistic Nursing*, Wiley, New York.
Pearson, A. (1988) Just an ordinary nurse, *Lakeside Graduation Address*, (unpublished).
Rieman, D.J. (1986) The essential structure of a caring interaction: doing phenomenology, in *Nursing Research: A Qualitative Perspective*. (eds P. Munhall and C.J. Oiler), Appleton-Century-Crofts, Norwalk.
Scheiermacher, F. (1977) *Hermeneutics: The Handwritten Manuscripts* (ed. H. Kimmerle and trans. J. Duke and J. Fortsman), Scholars Press, Atlanta.
Spiegelberg, H. (1970) On some human uses of phenomenology, in *Phenomenology in Perspective* (ed. F.J. Smith). Martinus Nijhoff, The Hague.
Spiegelberg, H. (1976) *The Phenomenological Movement*, Vols 1 and II, Martinus Nijhoff, The Hague.

Stapleton, T.J. (1983) *Husserl and Heidegger: The Question of a Phenomenological Beginning*, State University of New York Press, Albany.

Sukale, M. (1976) *Comparative Studies in Phenomenology*. Martinus Nijhoff, The Hague.

Taylor, B.J. (1988) What are the patients' perceptions of the usefulness of information given to them by nurses and what are the nurses' perceptions of their roles and constraints as teachers in giving effective patient education in a postnatal ward? A research paper submitted in partial fulfilment of the requirements for the degree of Master of Education, Deakin University, Geelong.

Van Kaam, A. (1959a) The nurse in the patient's world, *American Journal of Nursing*, **59** (12), pp. 1708–10.

Van Kaam, A. (1959b) Phenomenological analysis: Exemplified by a study of the experience of being really understood, *Individual Psychology*, **15**, pp. 66–72.

CHAPTER 9

Rethinking the survey

Allan Kellehear

INTRODUCTION

Is there a correct methodological approach to health research? Are there methods which are consistently superior for yielding valuable insights in comparison with other methods? I doubt it. In this chapter, I argue that methodological approaches have, or should have, little to do with brand loyalties or the convenience of one's usual skills in this area. Methodological choices should complement the research questions asked, as many a textbook will argue, but furthermore, the methods should also be sensitive to the needs and features of the respondents or social processes being studied.

In developing this line of thought, I will first spend some time contextualizing the debate about which methods are appropriate in social research. I will introduce the quantitative–qualitative debate and give a simple illustration of how research questions and subjects, away from the abstract debates, may determine a choice of methods. In the next section I will develop this theme with a major health example from my own research. Semi-structured interviewing with the dying, in a project aimed at surveying 100 terminally ill cancer sufferers is discussed. Common criticisms of surveys are fielded in this section to show how the research responded, not to favourite methodological dispositions, but rather to the unique circumstances and health of the respondents. I conclude that the survey method, that *enfant terrible* of qualitative researchers, deserves a rethink, especially if seen as a useful response to research with the very ill.

QUANTITATIVE VS. QUALITATIVE DEBATE

Mechanic (1989) has recently pointed out that the debate between methodological styles is still raging. People continue to argue the merits and demerits of positivism (which equates with quantitative and objective methods) and of naturalistic inquiry (which equates with qualitative and subjective methods). This philosophical–methodological split is part of a larger one in health sociology, indeed within health social sciences generally.

In historical terms one may trace this division to the Cartesian philosophical split. On the one hand, some assume that the world has a concrete reality separate from the personal experience of it. This is the view underpinning traditions such as positivism, empiricism and rationalism. On the other hand, the alternative subjectivist view argues that reality and one's experience of it are inseparable. Traditional advocates of this view can be found in existential, phenomenological and post-structuralist writings.

A variety of attitudes has been taken over this division, differences which have created much tension in health research discussions around the world. The first reaction has usually been to take sides in the debate, to develop a 'brand loyalty'. Here the quantitative people merely dismiss the qualitative approaches as unreliable and unrepresentative. The naturalistic, grounded theory-oriented researchers simply assert that survey methods have major validity problems. The post-structuralists go one step further by arguing that the concepts of reliability and validity belong to an empiricist discourse of dubious value. This style of language artificially elevates the researcher as a person able to make truth claims about the world which are assumed to be superior to those that he or she studies. Knowledge is about surveillance and power and debates about reliability and validity merely make sovereign, acts which are political rather than scientific.

Another reaction has been to take the magnanimous approach and attempt to be eclectic. Of course, this has usually necessitated turning a blind eye to post-structuralist concerns. One recommends a qualitative, thematic pilot study which will help generate emic categories, that is, categories which represent the native's point of view. From the findings of that pilot, one may then execute the more respectable and objective survey. As a methodological policy this is both uncritical and inflexible. As with the brand loyalty approach, this is a method rather than question-driven style of research work.

Another attitude, the one outlined by Mechanic (1989), is to understand that the theoretical and methodological divisions are responses to ambiguities about reality, truth, knowledge and experience. Away from the heat of debate, even semioticians will agree that 'even bad methods truly reveal' (Deely, 1990). Mechanic argues that **we** are the research tool and that the most important task is to calibrate ourselves. Most methods (ethnographic, semiotic or statistical) can be learnt by any monkey. How to use them to shed light, some small insight into questions you are asking, is the major challenge confronting investigators of human culture.

If you understand from the outset that you yourself (i.e. your questions, time constraints, resources, ethics, politics and so on) and those who participate in the research (their social and personal characteristics) are the main parameters, you might more easily resist the common temptation to feel superior or embarrassed because you are conducting qualitative or quantitative work. The task in conducting efficient and critical research is to learn that methods are simply a means to an end. And that 'end' is to develop some understanding about the social world. However Mechanic's article, advocating the imaginative 'calibration' of self, does not go far enough. Mechanic is concerned to emphasize a methodological approach which is both valid and reliable but also one that is true and closest to the world of the research participants. He does not discuss, and therefore does not demonstrate, how the participants themselves might shape the nature of the method used. He does not show how that influence from respondents might transcend the usual consideration of method based on theoretical notions of emic and etic, reliability and validity.

Mechanic does recognize that certain features of a group of respondents might affect the efficacy of a method. For example, flagging motivation and disinterest may be a problem for respondents who are asked to keep diaries about their health over long periods. He also recognizes that diary keeping is perhaps more suitable for the literate middle classes than for the working classes, or for those for whom English is a second language. But these are marginal to his central argument, though no doubt, not unimportant. My emphasis in this chapter, however, is to sketch this point in some detail. After a preliminary choice of method (will I employ interviews, document analysis and observations?), thinking about the type of respondents in any serious way will, or should on many occasions, be a greater influence on the methodological design than mere ideological preferences.

Before launching into a detailed health research example, let me provide a quick overview of the issues with a brief example. Rollo May (1967) is a psychologist with a deadline to meet.

> I sit home at my typewriter of a morning writing one of the chapters which follow in this book. As I work I experience myself as one who has to get a chapter done, who has set himself a deadline, who has patients coming this afternoon who he must be prepared to see beginning at two o'clock, and who must take some medicine to ward off a threatening cold. I glance up at the clock and I quickly count through the number of pages I have completed so far. As I write I find the uncomfortable thought pressing in, ''My colleague, Professor So-and-So, will not like this point; perhaps I should obfuscate my idea a little – make

it sound profound and not so easy to attack?'' I nobly ward off such an ignoble temptation; but I do shore up the defences of my argument, then pull myself away from the intruding thoughts and back to my typewriter. (1967)

There are a number of research questions which one could direct to the activity described by May (including, but leaving aside for the moment, my own identification with that passage). Among these questions might be:

1. How driven by deadlines and peer pressure are academics?
2. What social and psychological tensions exist for academics when they write professional papers?
3. What is academic freedom in the context of academic writing?

These three questions (and others you might think of) set the agenda. This sets the focus, creates the angle to be taken. This emphasis or perspective omits other interests or questions. A time–motion method might analyse the environmental constraints on May. A content analysis of that study might identify some of his professional values – more so if May kept a diary that we could get our hands on. In-depth interviews with a minimum of structure would discover other values and beliefs and might identify related attitudes or coping strategies. Letters, memos or memoirs might contextualize all this too. But as we get more imaginative with our methods, as we get a fuller and more exciting potential picture of May as an academic, and as our minds boggle at the wonderful possibility of an all out thick and thorough descriptive answer to our questions, we must finally anchor these ideas in real time, real person resources and constraints.

First, do we want to know or need to know **all** this to answer our main question? Might we gain some of this information more simply from past literature in this area? Second, how much time and financial resources do we have available for this project. Senior academics, particularly those with funding, may be able to shift the resource arithmetic their way, towards the ideal design. For the vast majority of postgraduate researchers, unfunded researchers, private researchers or researchers with tiny budgets, this will **not** be the case. Books which deconstruct the 'field experience' tell all too well how research is driven hard by practical rather than theoretical considerations. Finally, how much probing and intrusion will May, and other academics like him, tolerate and for what good reasons offered to them? In this context then, much research is about the broader arithmetic of ideals and reality. Theoretical and philosophical preferences divided by resource constraints, subtracted or perhaps multiplied by what respondents will tolerate or what their personal and social circumstances will permit. Too often, methodological discourse has concentrated on the theoretical, philosophical preferences and ideals. All too often, little discussion has revolved around how a method might suit a respondent more than a researcher. Post-structuralists are correct in that frequently decision making is dictated by the secret and self-affirming cultures of the researcher rather than the social features or needs of people that participate in the process. It is commonly **assumed** that the method that is most respondent friendly or facilitative to the respondent's world of meaning is the unstructured, grounded theory type interview. In the following example, I will demonstrate that sometimes a practical concern for the respondent can lead to an interesting, if not unexpected, use of a more traditional survey interview. And this, thoughtfully used, need not suffer from the traditional limitations commonly associated with it.

RESEARCH WITH DYING PEOPLE

When I reviewed the social research literature on death and dying I was rather surprised by the paucity of work examining the process of dying itself. More particularly very little work had been conducted that looked at the social process of dying from a dying person's point of view. Most of the little work in this particular area was problem-focused and caretaker oriented. By this I mean, that most social research on dying looked at the medical, psychological and social problems encountered by terminally ill people. Furthermore, interest tended to interrogate the caretaker view more so than the view of the actual people who were dying. Family and health professionals' views about, and reactions toward, dying people predominated. There were, of course, one or two popular works on the dying process but these were medical (Hinton, 1967) or psychologically oriented (Kubler-Ross, 1969). They were also quite old as studies. The final interesting feature about work on dying was that many of the studies used small samples, perhaps five or six people and up to 20 or 30 respondents. Aside from Kubler-Ross (1969) who interviewed 200 people for her study there was little attempt to gain a broader picture of conformity and a variety of social values and behaviour. And because Kubler-Ross did not provide a sample description it was almost impossible to see patterns of meaning or experiences which might be associated with gender or age or social class. These omissions in the literature became my research questions (Kellehear, 1990).

Returning to the May example, I asked those three questions which we applied to our hypothetical research into academics' work and life-style.

1. First, do I want to know or need to know **all** of this to answer my main question? In this case my main question was: What do people do and experience once they realize that they will die very soon?

What we are talking about, in asking that question, is attempting to sketch a general picture of a dying person's social life once they become aware that they are dying. Clearly I need to interview these people but what shall I ask?

2. How much time and financial resources do I have for this project? At least here the answer was reasonably clear. I had no funding for the project itself and I had to subsist on a post-graduate scholarship to keep body and soul together as well. Since this project would be the subject of my PhD work I estimated that I could afford to take between 12 and 24 months to complete the interviews (but preferably 12 months).
3. How much probing and intrusion will people who are terminally ill tolerate? And for what good reasons offered to them? In the end, this was the question that shaped the answers to the other two more than I could imagine.

Initial pilot interviews revealed that the people I chose to interview, cancer patients, had a good many physical problems. I had more time than they did in more ways than the obvious one. Many terminally ill people had trouble holding their concentration or controlling their pain, vomiting or nausea. Others found our discussions emotionally draining, as I too, often did. It became quickly apparent that the interviews should contain a high level of structure and be well focused. This helped those people whose concentration and memory were resources only to be captured with some effort. This also allowed the main work of the interview to be short and made more time for digression and support talk within the interview. Even so, the interviews took between one and two hours. Furthermore, if I was to interview reasonable numbers of dying people I also needed to sustain my own emotional ability to conduct the work. Talking and sitting with dying people and sharing their thoughts and feelings about life in general is very difficult work. The turnover and burnout experiences of hospice workers give ample warning to anyone underestimating the stress involved. I needed to seriously consider the possiblity of personally 'burning out' before the research was completed. If I insisted on talking to 100 dying people I would need (1) a high rate of participation and (2) an ability to structure an interview for maximum support for both the interviewer and the person being interviewed.

The participation rate was high – only four refused out of 104. I simply told people that the social story of dying had not been told and I was hoping to do this. People were very keen to help and, despite the many painful and funny moments that we shared, most of the respondents found the exercise worthwhile for their own reasons. I have discussed these experiences in terms of research ethics elsewhere (Kellehear, 1989).

Structure in interviews, particularly imposed structures of the traditional survey interview, have been the subject of several criticisms, especially from qualitative researchers. I was aware of that criticism but I was faced with a group of people with special needs. How, within this professional tension, was I to overcome the emic–etic problem in this context. If I was to 'structure' the interview in traditional survey interview format whose categories would I use to perform this?

Combing the historical and anthropological literature I regularly came across the idea of the Good Death. The Good Death was a phrase described in a variety of countries (Western and non-Western) which described dying in terms of how the dying person and his or her community expected dying to occur. As one flips through the various accounts of dying from Victorian England to the Kaliai in Western New Britain several patterns repeatedly emerged. These patterns reflected the recurring cares and concerns of dying people themselves – awareness of dying, social adjustments, preparations for death, work disengagement and saying farewell. Depending on **how** each of these was performed one could gain an idea of the pressures and expectations on the dying, whilst often the dying themselves simply viewed each of these concerns as uniquely personal.

Although an unorthodox way of obtaining emic categories, I used these areas of concern to structure the interview questions: Who told you that you are dying? How did you discover this? What adjustments are you making for the pain or treatment side effects? How has this affected your relationships? What preparations have you made for the prospect of your death? Will you remain at work? Why? Why not? Will you say goodbye to anyone? Who? How? or Why not? There were many refinements and further questions developed to 'operationalize' the ideas behind the interview schedule. Furthermore, some question areas were more difficult than others. Questions concerning farewells for example, consistently aroused emotion and so these were asked toward the end of the interview. The less taxing, 'lighter weight' demographic questions which are commonly asked at the beginning of interviews, were instead located after the farewell questions. This provided all of us with a short relief from the task of intellectual and emotional reflection and recall. Also because of the ease with which these could be answered, more time could be spent here in supportive conversation and debriefing – the demographic questions could be answered during a coffee or light conversation.

The following are the most common concerns about using a traditional survey interview. First, since surveys are quick and less invasive they can be seen as superficial and non-involving. Second, since it was semi-structured, the interviews impose structures rather than allowing these to emerge. Finally, survey interviews are positivistic methods and they therefore imply either atheoretical approaches or theoretical ones which are ahistorical and functionalist (conservative in politics and sociological imagination). Let me, by way of prompting a rethink about survey interviews, answer each of these equally traditional criticisms in the context of my work with the dying.

Quick and less invasive equals superficial and non-involving

Quickness does not lead logically to superficiality. Superficiality is about the poor quality of an interview relationship. However, my research with the dying was hardly door-stop, door-step surveying but a non-medical, life review discussion. Non-involvement is only partly true in this context. An exchange of emotions and ideas is common in a short time. The issue of personal dying tends to draw people toward intense and mutual sharing. Anyone who has sat with a friend for an hour talking about their marriage break-up or grief over the death of a friend will recognize this much. It is difficult to be superficial if the topics themselves are not superficial. Superficiality is reasonably easy in a 10-minute exchange but becomes progressively more difficult if the time is increased and if the conversation turns from abstract topics to highly personal ones.

Nevertheless, one-and-a-half hours is not one-and-a-half days or one-and-a-half years. This level of involvement is not desirable either for the respondent or for the interviewer. The interviewer needs a certain level of personal distance to facilitate a prolonged stay in conducting this work. Also, long interviews tax cancer sufferers considerably, particularly toward the end of their illness. Follow-up interviews or double checking interpretations of the transcripts are often not possible. Many respondents died several days or weeks later, making these kinds of practices impossible to conduct. Only the healthier and more tolerant cancer sufferer would be available for this kind of approach.

Imposed categories inferior to inductive ones

The interview categories used were not simply 'invented' by me. As I mentioned earlier, the central categories were adopted from phenomenological sources in history, anthropology and even creative literature. Too frequently, sceptics of the survey feel that since survey categories are commonly etic ones that this feature of the survey cannot be changed. Or if change is possible, unstructured interviews should be the stimulus for that change. I am suggesting that emic categories can actually be gleaned from past social science literature as well.

However, I recognize that these categories may not be as emic as I believe. But it is useful to remember at this juncture that the interview was semi-structured and allowed respondents significant opportunity to develop their own narratives. Furthermore, the first question and one of the final questions was more general, open and facilitative of their own narratives. The first question asked was: What do you believe is the single most important change in your life since the onset of your illness? This is similar to a 'critical incident' type question often used in personal construct psychology. The final question was: Can you describe any aspect of your life which has undergone minor or major changes as a consequence of your illness and the prospect that you might die, which we have not so far discussed?

Furthermore, not much significance can be logically attached to omissions if one was to use an 'unstructured' interview because memory or recall is hindered by pain, illness or deep fatigue. In any case, unstructured interviews are no less prone to shaping responses. One's sex, occupation, personality or physical/social appearance can influence responses, stimulating people to answer in certain ways or along certain lines of thought.

Whether interviews are structured, semi-structured or unstructured is no indication or guarantee in itself of the reliability or the validity of the findings. Interview categories may be shared by the culture of the respondents. Narrative analysis may impose 'themes' which are truer for interviewer than for interviewee. Kubler-Ross (1969) for example, employed unstructured interviews with over 200 terminally ill people to 'inductively' develop a stage theory of dying – a theory no one else has been able to substantiate to date.

Survey methods atheoretical or at least ahistorical

This is an ironic criticism in a way. It is designed, to borrow an American vaudeville line, 'never to give a sucker an even break'. In other words, surveys are bad methods if they are atheoretical and bad if they imply a theory. This is an example of a criticism designed to protect its own survival. The object of the criticism has no escape – damned if it does, damned if it does not (have a theory). In the specific example of research with the dying, the theoretical approach was both historical and phenomenological. It was historical because the main features of dying were extrapolated from contemporary, cross-cultural and historical sources. Furthermore, how these features emerged or expressed themselves within my sample of dying people was connected to the social and political interest of the day. The rise of professions, the work ethic and the gradual distancing and alienation of family units from their economic means of production was linked to the meanings, behaviours and experiences of today's dying. A view of dying, from the dying person's perspective, was used as a guide to these changes, developments and issues.

This was no conservative political or sociological account. In any case methodological approaches are not a reliable indicator. Methods do not necessarily imply theories nor do certain theories necessarily dictate certain methods. When C. Wright Mills (1959) wrote about the sociological imagination he was not confining his remarks to theory. He referred to the whole enterprise of social investigation and explanation and that includes method. His comments are no less true today than before. The practical project drives the method and it alone provides the main social, ethical and bureaucratic constraints and parameters within which the researcher must work.

Let me summarize the main influences which shaped the methodological style and outcomes of my enquiry with dying cancer sufferers. First, the poor nature of their health prompted me to look for a less invasive style of method (e.g. not observations, not in-depth interviews). Second, the nature of these constraints prompted me to look elsewhere for themes or question areas other than pursuing this in early unstructured interviews. Third, not having unlimited or even long respondent time available forced me to think seriously about how much information I really needed to develop a basic social picture of dying. This suggested that I should 'economize my general curiosity' rather than ask as much about everything that the respondent was capable of answering. This is another prompt for some prior organization and structure in any interviewing to be done. Finally, the process of identifying and gaining permission from each terminal cancer sufferer and then arranging the interview and then actually conducting the interview before they became too ill or died made the whole process take about 15 months. Both the type of people I wished to interview and the sheer and simple arithmetic of their availability, rather than any of my own aims or ideals, determined the length of time to complete the project. I did interview 100 people – an important requirement if the results were to be of interest to the sea of positivists which is the medical profession, however a trifle irrelevant to qualitative methodologists in the social sciences. Since I was hoping to make some modest contribution to the care of dying people as well as to sociology in general, I was influenced by both the medical and sociological discourses about method.

RETHINKING THE SURVEY

I began this chapter by sketching a brief overview of the qualitative-quantitative debate. In the theory of method literature at least, the main arguments revolved around which methods are best in terms of reliability/validity and emic/etic issues. Rarely however do these factors solely determine one's choice of method. The practical constraints of the researcher's resources often determine choice of method and how many or how few are used. Furthermore, little discussion has highlighted how the social and personal features of the people investigated might best determine the type of method used. The use of survey interviews in health research is a fine example of this point. Despite qualitative wisdom to the contrary, structured survey interviews have the potential to be just as 'respondent friendly' and emically sound as less structured interviews which permit greater narrative analysis. In certain circumstances then, the decision to use the former over the latter is taken because the survey interview is able to maintain these features even in the face of interviewing the very ill respondent. Research with the dying illustrates exactly how this is so. From a review of that research, we may conclude the following.

Reliability and validity are not the only considerations in choosing a method. The people investigated by the study also play a significant part in the selection and this, as in my case example, can be quite significant. It may lead to the use of a survey method, it may not, but the nature of the people one is interested in studying should help decide rather than simply one's personal philosophical preferences.

There is nothing intrinsically determinist about the features of a survey. Highly structured or highly unstructured interviews are not intrinsically ahistorical, less valid or theoretically impoverished. If the categories and questions used are not derived from the respondent this does not necessarily mean that the instrument is less valid, or hopelessly lost and alienated from the world of the respondent. The researcher is not always, and by biblical definition, a bringer of etic meaning. Past literature can sensitize where personal biography limits. Empathy, understanding and identification with others have many sources; and some of these may emerge in a narrative analysis and others may materialize through contact with a wide range of creative and scientific literature.

The quick and structured nature of a survey interview can be a positive advantage to those with less time or for whom the passage of time is complicated by distracting physical and social demands. Depth and quality of an exchange is associated with rapport and trust rather than simply whether interviews are more or less structured. More structure and brevity of an interview can make analysis a little more difficult but these features are ethically more considerate and suitable for some types of respondents, particularly very ill people.

Brand loyalties in methodological discourse have their advantages in terms of in-group loyalties, professional identity formation and status. However, choosing methods outside these can occasionally have benefits for the respondents without necessarily sacrificing validity or emic considerations. Furthermore, using other methods may make contributions to other discourse outside our own by using less favoured methods more imaginatively. This creates interest from those in other discourses despite the temporary stigma and disapproval one may receive from one's usual associates. Finally, are there groups or circumstances, aside from dying, which might make one think about using a simple structured or semi-structured survey? In light of the preceding experience and discussion I think that this is a fair and appropriate question to pose. Health research is commonly conducted with and by people who enjoy reasonable physical health. However, research with the very old, the chronically ill and the acutely ill is increasing, partly at least, because the epidemiological picture in industrial societies is shifting in this direction. But the desire by many researchers for time-consuming, unstructured conversations may not sit well or be easily accommodated by these populations of sick people.

Given that constraint, and put in that context, the survey may well do with being reconsidered occasionally. In this way, we may rehabilitate an old and common method and put it to new use.

REFERENCES

Deely, J. (1990) *Basics of Semiotics*, Indiana University Press, Bloomington.
Hinton, J. (1967) *Dying*, Penguin, Harmondsworth.
Kellehear, A. (1989) Ethics and social research, in *Doing Fieldwork: Eight Personal Accounts of Social Research* (J. Perry), Deakin University Press, Geelong.
Kellehear, A. (1990) *Dying of Cancer: The Final Year of Life*, Harwood Academic Publishers, London.
Kubler-Ross, E. (1969) *On Death and Dying*, Macmillan, New York.
May, R. (1967) *Psychology and the Human Dilemma*, Van Nostrand, New York.
Mechanic, D. (1989) Medical Sociology: Some tensions among theory, method and substance, *Journal of Health and Social Behaviour* **30**, pp. 147–60.
Mills, C. Wright (1959) *The Sociological Imagination*, Oxford University Press, New York.

CHAPTER 10

Evaluating drug education programmes

Rob Walker

Evaluation is increasingly a requirement of any interventive or action programme in health, education and elsewhere. Outside the USA it has grown from being the minority interest of a few specialists to an integral concern for any specially funded project or programme. An informal survey sent out to drug educators attending two major conferences in Australia during 1989, revealed a growing awareness and some unease at the prospect of increasing demands on projects and programmes for evaluation reports of one kind or another.

GOOD REASONS FOR BEING WARY OF EVALUATION

The need for evaluation is often stated but rarely argued. The demands an evaluation makes are almost always derived from the needs of those in the bureaucracy; those responsible for distributing funds want information on costs, activities and consequences. An evaluation may be required or requested in the name of the public interest but invariably it is framed in terms of the management needs of the system.

Evaluation can serve useful educational functions. It can be the most effective way in which a programme learns about itself and records what it has learnt for others but increasingly this formative function is frequently eclipsed by the needs of managers who need to know how money is being spent.

The purpose of an evaluation study is to provide information to those who are in positions where they can influence specific policies or practices in forms and at times which will cause them to question their judgement. By definition evaluation is a political activity. It may involve some research activities and aspire to promote research as an element of professional practice but, in itself, it is both more and less than research – more, in that it is interventive and needs to be acutely aware of its own role within the settings in which it acts, and less, in that the claims it makes will always be localized and specific.

There are many good reasons for wanting to evaluate drug education programmes and most of them seem at first sight to be unproblematic. Of course, so conventional rhetoric argues, it would be a good idea to know more about the effectiveness of programmes, about their costs, difficulties and triumphs; for it is only in that way can we improve services, learn from others, and get the best value for money. The better the information we have, it is often argued, the better will be the quality of the services that we provide.

If life were so simple there would be no drug problem. What appears at first glance to be rational and self-evidently worthwhile is not always so in practice. Evaluation, like drug use, has its dark side. What is set out in words of reason can become an instrument of control, designed to prevent innovation rather than encouraging it. Those who commission evaluations often do so to pre-empt action and to deflect critical comment.

This sounds faintly paranoid but evaluation does not need conspiracies, for it can be its own worst enemy. The limited range of techniques, methods and objectives adopted by evaluators can get in the way, set their own priorities, create their own distractions and be used by evaluators merely to further their own careers. It is not that evaluators are any more prone to corruption than anyone else, but that the nature of their work takes them into places where research tends not to venture. Researchers are relatively free to set their own agenda but evaluations are invariably commissioned by the relatively powerful into the work that the less powerful do to improve the lot of the relatively powerless. Evaluation is a social process, frequently accompanied by a moral mission, and it follows that corruption is endemic, not necessarily in the narrow monetary sense, but in the sense that independence is extraordinarily difficult to maintain in the face of close relationships.

With the best of intentions, an evaluation can make practical action more difficult to achieve. The process of decision making, for example, is not necessarily improved by being fully and adequately informed. The result may be to stall the process as those concerned become overwhelmed with information and paralysed by understanding. Evaluation is primarily concerned to ask questions, and not to provide answers, which can make life uncomfortable and frustrating for those whose job it is to optimize the provision of solutions to problems given to them by others.

Given the difficulties, what is it reasonable to expect of an evaluation? First, we should be clear that an evaluation is always and only an evaluation of a programme. We cannot evaluate generalizations and abstractions. It is reasonable to attempt to evaluate **this** programme with **this** staff, **these** resources, in **these** circumstances. It is not possible to evaluate general and pervasive categories like 'methadone programmes', 'early intervention' or 'social skills'. A programme which is differently staffed or supported in other circumstances at another time and place may realize quite different outcomes. Evaluation, by definition, is always about specifics, never about generalities. In this sense it is very different from experimental research, which may well seek to make such claims by conceptually discarding specific effects in order to focus on what may be claimed to be generalizable in a programme.

Second, evaluation always needs to be concerned with **whole** programmes. In itself the measurement of variables and effects provides only limited and partial understanding. In evaluating programmes we have, necessarily, to take into account a wide range of concerns; we have to consider what Stake (1967) has called the 'countenance' of evaluation. We have to ask questions, not just about effects, but about process, history, context and biography. The responsibility of the evaluator, in Stake's (1972) words is to provide 'portrayal' rather than 'analysis'.

Perhaps the greatest difficulty most of us have is with the role of judgement in relation to evaluation. Following the points I have just made it might seem reasonable to expect the evaluator to make judgements about the quality or worth of specific programmes, acting as a broker between what is publicly known about the field of action and the performance of a particular programme. Certainly one popular image and a common expectation is of the evaluator providing judgement on programmes, but the notion of singular professional judgement is increasingly difficult to sustain in almost any field. Many evaluators prefer to see themselves in what Barry MacDonald (1974), an experienced British evaluator, has called an 'honest broker role'. In most social action programmes (and drug education is certainly no exception) almost any action is contentious; programme staff and evaluators quickly find themselves entering realms of conflicting social values. What is the role of the evaluator in such circumstances? The answer MacDonald gives is that the task of the evaluator is to locate and clarify issues, to foster debate and to provide relevant and accurate information: not to offer judgement, but to collect judgements, to examine them and to juxtapose them in an attempt to create balanced accounts.

To take this role is to amplify the political significance of the evaluation, for the evaluator comes to know a lot about the people, perspectives and events that make up the work of the project, even when operating within strict and disciplined procedures (as advocated, for instance, by MacDonald 1974; MacDonald and Walker, 1974; Kemmis and Robottom, 1981). Despite procedural neutrality the evaluator can become influential within the programme. Many evaluators have been surprised to find that actions that they intended to be neutral and minimally interventive are not seen as such by those being evaluated. Even the interview, often seen as a relatively benign instrument, can be powerfully interventionist and more influential in bringing about change than directives from the central office.

Given the highly charged environments within which evaluations are usually conducted, arriving at a workable set of procedures can become a key concern for evaluators. In trying to sort out some of these complexities, MacDonald offers a typology which is political in its perspective and distinguishes 'democratic', 'autocratic' and 'bureaucratic' forms of evaluation. What is important to note is that the focus here is not on methods so much as on situated ethics. The prime concern is to find satisfactory grounds for the relationships evaluators should have with programme personnel, participants and clients, given that these people occupy positions which give them differential access to power.

MacDonald's preferred approach he defines, provocatively, as 'democratic'. Its concern, he argues, is to provide information to all those involved or concerned with a programme, irrespective of their status or role. Whatever the precepts and expectations or the organizations involved, the democratic evaluator treats clients and staff on an equal footing with sponsors and administrators. The evaluation model allows for no privileged access, disavows the use of specialist language and technical data and writes its reports for a general audience. In contrast, 'bureaucratic' evaluation is a service provided for administrators and officials. They pay for it, the report is for them and they judge both the programme and the evaluation. Its language and style may well be technical and will be restricted both in its codes and in its intended readership. An 'autocratic' evaluation shades into research, for it draws on the authority of the researcher, trusting him or her to ask the right questions and provide appropriate answers. The key audience is seen to be the academic peer group, the style and presentation frequently adopting the conventions of the academy.

It is important not to confuse the 'democratic' and the 'bureaucratic' in evaluation for to do so is to confuse significant differences of purpose and intent. To engage in evaluation is to deal in the transfer of information; information being the currency of power in such circumstances. As a shorthand, any time we find ourselves involved in evaluation we need to ask ourselves:

- Who is it for?
- What will be the consequences?

- Who gains and who loses?
- Who learns most?

The questions sound simple, but the answers rarely are and, almost always, they have significant implications and consequences.

THE DRUG EDUCATION PROBLEM

It is hard to avoid the fact that non-medical drug use presents a major contemporary social problem. Read any newspaper, in any country in the world, and the chances are that you will find a prominent drug story, and the news is invariably bad. A major drug seizure gets headline treatment; a prominent sporting figure is barred from competition; drug-related violent crime is identified as linked with police corruption.

As drug stories have become a dependable theme in the minds of newspaper and magazine editors, so politicians looking for press attention will tell their speech writers to address the 'war against drugs' (Bell, 1975; Beniger, 1983). The modern urban myths that they draw upon include the themes that drugs are associated with the life-styles of the rich and famous, that truck drivers use drugs to stay awake, that drugs are commonly used in both professional and amateur sport and that drugs are sold and used in schools. True or untrue, so regular and persistent are the stories that their messages have become part of the backdrop to modern life. What does this mean for education? In particular what does it mean for those who teach or work in schools?

The shift of attention to the role of schools appears to have come about because other professions are seen to have failed, rather than because schools have positive solutions to offer. The political and policy response to the problems that arise from drug abuse has been passed, successively, from law and law enforcement, to medicine, health, social work, therapy, advertising and, increasingly, to the schools. This has paralleled a successive shift from the hope that drug abuse can be eradicated, to a view that it can be treated, that it can be prevented, that it can be controlled.

The usual first response of governments to the drug problem is to adopt legal prohibition, a move that is often modified through a series of policies that are referred to as 'supply control' strategies. As a first response to the problem this seems rational, but in practice it rarely works as intended because the real problem is often very different to the espoused problem. 'Supply control' has been found to have some effect in controlling the use of legal drugs (the use of alcohol and tobacco by young people in particular) but little effect in controlling illegal drug use. Indeed the introduction of harsh penalties for possession of such drugs may have been in the interests of organized crime and those officials engaged in corruption, for the main effect has been to create a market with a high value-added component.

Whatever the reasons, the emphasis of those in policy positions (as marked in particular by recent White House statements on the drug problem) has been to look to 'demand control'. President Bush singled out the important role the schools should play, while others have been content to advocate even simpler solutions. 'Just say No', said Nancy Reagan, to be echoed by the Australian Life Education Programme in one of its publicity campaigns.

What are the consequences for the schools, now that the problem has been handed to them? The law has failed, the police have failed, social workers and therapists of various persuasions have failed. What is it reasonable to expect schools and teachers to be able to do?

In the UK and Australia, the response has been a curriculum response. What we have seen in the last six or seven years has been a flowering of curricula in the form of kits, tapes, posters, videos, games and training programmes. Go to any conference on drug education and you will find a space set aside for people to display their wares, and most of them are well produced, attractive and well thought out. In the classroom, most of it works. Those who have sponsored and produced material include ministry curriculum staff, the Quit campaign, the road traffic authorities, the pharmacists' professional association, police, educational publishers and the Life Education Programme.

Looking at this material a number of things stand out:

- The problem is clearly identified as lying with legal rather than illegal drugs.
- A predominant emphasis is on developing social, personal and decision-making skills among students.
- Three key audiences are identified: primary school-aged children, for general drug education programmes; 16 and 17 year-old males for drink–driving programmes; early adolescence (especially girls) for smoking prevention programmes.

Why the emphasis on legal rather than illegal drugs? One of the things that has happened to the drug problem as it has been passed from law enforcement to health professionals is that the problem itself has been transformed in important ways. This is especially true in Australia, as well as in the UK and some other European countries. This shift in emphasis in the way that the drug problem is defined, away from illegal to legal drug use, marks a dramatic shift in thinking which has considerable implications for teachers and educators faced with what looks to be an intractable problem. It has been brought about by the efforts of a relatively small group of health researchers and health professionals, particularly in the UK and Australia.

For teachers, educators and schools, basing a drug education programme on the dangers of legal drugs means that rather than simply reinforcing a message that most parents will share, teachers find themselves taking a point of view that puts them in conflict with attitudes and values that are an implicit part of the culture. When President Bush (among others) said that he saw schools as being in the 'front-line of the War Against Drugs' he did not know the significance of the remark. For teachers to engage in drug education means putting themselves into an area marked by contentious social values. It means running against the grain of many media assumptions and it means putting their own ways of life up for scrutiny, often in the face of hostility from other teachers, parents and the community. This issue is sharpened in a context where policy initiatives stress the needs for schools to be responsive to their communities, and where parents in particular may be placed in positions where they can directly influence decisions about curriculum and school organization.

As curriculum decisions become more politicized, one of the first things teachers need to ask themselves when they take on drug education, is whether they are more likely to be part of the problem than part of the answer. They have to examine their own patterns and habits of drug use, perhaps even their own dependencies. They have to ask themselves what models they provide and attempt to identify what forms of resistance they are likely to provoke in their students.

CURRICULUM OR SCHOOLING?

I mentioned earlier that the way education has responded to being handed the drug problem has been to develop curricula. This solves the immediate practical problem of knowing what to do but it is not without its difficulties, especially in secondary schools. The initial problems of deciding what to teach, to whom, when and how, are quickly followed by further questions. Where is it to be placed in the timetable? Who will teach it? Will it be assessed? There is little uniformity in the answers that schools have devised for these problems and little shared experience among teachers. Given the variations and short life of most programmes, some evaluators have concentrated on the problem of describing what is happening, to the frustration of others who see value only in measured differences in the short-term between pre- and post-tests of attitude and behaviour.

The question we have almost all avoided is whether schools are able to bring about the kinds of transformation in attitudes, values and behaviour in the long-term that seems to be demanded. In making policy decisions we seem to have fallen for our rhetoric, believing that schools are educational institutions that act rationally to achieve their goals, aims and objectives. But paradoxically, if you were asked to design settings which might encourage drug use among young people, schools would seem to provide optimum conditions. Schools provide an environment in which drug taking is prohibited or disapproved by adult authority and surrounded by the weight of institutional sanction, yet they often act informally to celebrate drug use as an adult social convention.

Schools and colleges provide the ground for close peer relationships, social networks and activities and an implicit culture of deception and risk-taking that appears designed to support a culture of resistance. The fact is that in the adult community, drug use is associated with relaxation and desirable life-styles (motor racing, team sports and rock music for example), yet schools both deny these things to the young and deny adulthood to the adolescent. This leads me to suggest that it would not be surprising to find that, behind the facade of the formal curriculum, schools in fact act to encourage the very thing that they deny. The source of the drug 'problem' may not lie in the peer group but in the institution of schooling.

Despite the well-meaning efforts that have been put into curriculum development, from a teacher's perspective the problem would appear to be less with the curriculum than with the hidden curriculum. One of the few things we know about the hidden curriculum is that any attempts we make to manipulate or control it are likely to lead to surprising outcomes and even to reversals of our aims and intentions.

Looking deeper into the nature and structure of schooling in order to explain the insistence that students are not adult, it would seem that part of the educational problem for schools and colleges stems from their dual role, and frequent confusion between being educational in intent but custodial in practice. In this context, an issue like drug use takes on many complications. As well as a public expectation that they act as agencies for moral and social control, schools have an affinity, perhaps derived from their historical origins, for moralizing and rhetoric that often undoes their best intentions of acting educationally.

The problem for schools is that they stand on a knife edge, acting at one moment for the parents and at the next for the state. Teachers are frequently caught between their desire to act as agents of socialization, and the requirement that they act as agents of institutionalization. Their role is both to educate and to control but their vocation also demands that they enter into relationships with their students. You do not have to watch *Dead Poets' Society* to know that this can be a dangerous and uncomfortable place.

STRATEGIES IN THE FACE OF AN IMPOSSIBLE TASK

If the drug problem calls on schools for a response that they cannot provide, what should be the task of an evaluation? If the problem demands a response that is more complex and subtle than can be met by our desire to create curriculum packages and training programmes, should an evaluation confine itself to evaluating those materials against the aims and objectives that they set for themselves?

Drug education provides a case that exemplifies the fact that it is not enough to evaluate a programme and its performance against its own declared aims and objectives. To do so does not allow for fallibility in either the policy or the proposal in a field where failure is virtually inevitable. In any curriculum development, those who designed the programme should have the opportunity to realize the limitations of their own understanding of the effects and consequences of their actions. They need to be given freedom to fail on condition that they learn from their errors of judgement.

Critical appraisal of the aims and objectives in terms of their relevance and appropriateness is an important element in any evaluation, and one which forces the evaluator to confront the politics of educational values that lie at the heart of any educational programme.

It is not enough for a programme to claim that it has met its objectives. It may be more important to ask whether or not these objectives are worthwhile and appropriate, whether the programme has made a clear analysis of its potential to bring about change and whether it has made intelligent decisions and understands its limitations, dysfunctions and shortfalls. In the long run what may be most important in any programme is not what is achieved but what has been learnt. A programme may be best judged, not by its outcomes, but by what those people who are involved in it do next. The evaluation task is, in large part, to help people redefine what counts as success.

I can understand why some evaluators see their task as identifying behavioural outcomes from drug programmes, arguing that it is only programmes that demonstrably make a difference that can be said to be effective. Yet we know that short-term gains, in this sense, are often illusory. When we are talking about children and young adolescents, an attitude, value or behaviour that appears to be established at one point in time may be so context-bound that a change in context triggers a later block or reversal. We probably all know of young children strongly opposed to smoking who later become tobacco users, and secondary students who reward themselves for writing an essay on the dangers of smoking by smoking a cigarette. As Roger Barker (1968) showed many years ago, behaviour is powerfully shaped by ecology, a point developed with an action orientation to health issues by Kickbusch (1988, 1989). As young people move from school to college or school to unemployment or school to work, the new contexts in which they find themselves are likely to be more powerful in bringing about behavioural change than anything we do in a short classroom-based programme.

What we need is a better understanding of the settings within which action is embedded. To understand drug use in schools we need to understand the schools, and change them, just as much as we need to understand the student-as-user. Adding drug education to an already overloaded curriculum is not likely to have major effects so long as the curriculum itself remains competitive, academic and boring.

What an educational evaluation can do is to ask questions, rather than limiting its role to giving answers. It can make connections between a specific programme in a particular school and the experience others might have had elsewhere. Descriptions of instances and cases can provide a basis for developing shared and continuing experience. Description is important but it is not enough. Evaluation has to go beyond description if it is to ask questions about the strategies that are adopted and the choices that are made, even implicitly, between one set of actions and another.

In teaching about drugs as in teaching about anything else, much has to be taken on trust, and in relation to such questions, evaluation does not always help. Yet, in an area that is inherently so difficult we need evaluation if we are to accumulate any basis for future wisdom. The primary need is for description related to analysis and critical comment. Measuring effectiveness is an illusion.

It was with these thoughts in mind that I turned to the problem of evaluating a drug education programme using case studies. For the past six years I have been involved in evaluating the Education Programme of Geelong Centre for Alcohol and Drug Dependence, a one-person programme evaluated by a fractional evaluator. The aim of the case studies we have produced has been to create the basis for discussion of the issues and encourage the development of an evaluation culture among teachers and others.

The case studies we have written and researched have an opening section which describes our intent:

Intentions
These reports are not intended to provide recommendations but to improve professional judgement. Many schools face the

problems and difficulties of introducing drug education, each school is different and each has its own story to tell. In this series of research studies we attempt to tell some of those stories.

Our intention is to set down a record of each school's experience in the area of drug education to give the reader access to the actions, thoughts and reflections of those who have been directly involved in drug education programmes. Our belief is that reporting in this way we may be able to avoid the recurrent curriculum problem of having to reinvent and rediscover successful strategies each time a school attempts an intervention into the existing curriculum. Perhaps more important, in an area of curriculum reform that is necessarily so difficult and publicly sensitive, we need to be aware of what might go wrong. Knowing the mistakes that others have made, if we understand their actions fully, can perhaps save us from making similar mistakes.

The cases we intend to report will not be selected because anyone claims them to be outstanding successes or abject failures. As far as possible we will report the experiences of 'ordinary' schools, attempting to accomplish something we know to be very difficult within constraints of resources and human capabilities we think most readers will recognize and acknowledge.

Origins
We began this series as part of the evaluation of a drug education programme. In 1985 the Geelong Centre for Alcohol and Drug Dependence appointed Margaret Clark to a new position as Education Officer. The proposal to establish this position included an evaluation element.

The first case studies in this series tried to assess the impact of the Centre's programme by examining developments in schools where Margaret had worked. Our aim was to see what happened after Margaret had left, rather than looking closely at what she did, and in this way providing her with some means of assessing the effectiveness of different intervention strategies.

The purpose of evaluation
As the series has continued, the focus on the Centre's programme has diminished. We have continued to focus on schools with which Margaret has had contact, but the schools themselves, their programmes and their problems have loomed larger in the case studies than the Centre's programme. The uninformed reader might find it difficult to see how the more recent case studies constitute an evaluation of the programme.

We would still claim that they do! We believe that the purpose of programme evaluation is to provide information that can form the basis of improved judgement. In going beyond the scope of the drug education officer's immediate work to examine the contexts within which she works, we are able to provide her and the Centre with some sense of the limited scope of their actions. We believe an evaluation should not simply hold performance up against a set of objectives, but should ask whether or not people have acted intelligently in the face of daunting and complex issues. In evaluating the work of the Centre it is important to ask questions about the judgements that have been made about how, when and where to offer support (and when not to).

This explains why these case studies include only a limited account of the immediate work of the programme. It also explains why the focus is wider than a concern with the immediate 'drug education' curriculum.

In looking at drug education programmes in schools we quickly learnt that behind the appearance of 'drug education' as an item in the syllabus or a label on the timetable lay a complex web of interrelated issues. How was that timetable space created? Who was teaching it? To which classes at what level? These, and similar questions, led us to ask more general questions about school organization and policy: questions that other schools attempting to introduce simlar courses would need to answer. At its simplest: to introduce a new course means, not only that someone has to be found to teach it, but at the cost of someone not teaching something else.

Rob Walker
Deakin University
March, 1990

We have written case studies intended for a broad readership in the hope that we could create 'a community of knowledgeable users'. In practice the cases have mostly been read and used by other evaluators and researchers – another case to validate the Fox hypothesis. (This derives from the American evaluator, Tom Fox, who has claimed that the degree to which an evaluation has an impact on practice is a function of personal and professional investment in the evaluation process. It follows that, since the greatest investment is made by the evaluators, it is the evaluator's practice that is most changed by the evaluation.)

This gives rise to a central dilemma for evaluation in the face of contentious programmes for, on the one hand, there is a strong case to be made for evaluation being independent, and carried out by people who are formally and actually disconnected from the programme.

On the other hand, the stronger the boundary between the programme and the evaluation, the less investment the programme will have in the evaluation and the less it will change their approach to the task.

Some programmes have managed this difficulty by adopting a strategy which combines formal independence and informal inter-action and involvement. Typically this involves a structured set of procedures for managing the communication of evaluation reports but close personal and social interaction with all programme participants. The risks involved in this strategy are high and the survival skills required of the evaluator very demanding.

Another possible strategy is to merge the evaluation role with responsibility for dissemination, action research and training. This approach is often favoured by administrators and policy-makers because it reduces the threat of critical comment posed by an inde-pendent evaluation and brings the evaluation itself within the grasp of the programme. The danger for the evaluator is exactly the same, in that the need to produce action often drowns out the need to establish a critical voice. Many early curriculum development projects (for example most of the projects supported by the Schools Council in the UK during the 1970s) adopted this approach and found themselves with evaluations that were compromised on key issues and ineffective and lacking in credibility when external audiences began to question the worth of the programmes.

For those involved in evaluating programmes the decisions that need to be made about the role of the evaluation are not simply method-ological but ethical and political. The evaluation of any programme should take within its scope the evaluation of policy as well as the evaluation of performance. It is not enough to judge performance against objectives that are not in themselves questioned, indeed interrogation of policy objectives may be the central function of an independent evaluation. One of the unacknowledged strengths of case study methods is their capacity to move between levels of a pro-gramme, that is to ask both whether those in policy-making positions have made intelligent decisions and to ask what happens to these decisions in practice. To accomplish this means redefining what counts as a 'case', as an issue or concern that cuts across organizational levels within a programme. This requires an imaginative leap, for the traditions that evaluation tends to draw on (usually using the language of 'ethnography' but the ideas and practice of symbolic interaction) have deeply inscribed into their assumptions the belief that face-to-face interaction is where social structure is to be found. Stepping beyond this assumption to include bureaucratic structures and inter-action that may be as much based in the literary as the spoken word, presents a considerable challenge.

ACKNOWLEDGEMENTS

The paper derives from an evaluation of the Education Programme at the Geelong Centre for Alcohol and Drug Dependence. A detailed account of the history of the programme and some case studies of schools are available from the Deakin Institute for Studies in Education, Deakin University, Victoria 3217. Some of the ideas outlined here are being further developed in the context of an ARC funded project, 'Schooling the Future' based at Deakin and involving Richard Bates, Chris Bigum, Lindsay Fitzclarence, Bill Green, Meredith O'Neil and Karen Tregenza.

REFERENCES

Barker, R. (1968) *Ecological Psychology: Concepts and Methods for Studying the Environment of Human Behaviour*, Stanford University Press, Stanford.

Bell, P. (1975) Drugs and the media, *Australian Alcohol and Drug Review*, **42** (2), pp. 235–42.

Collins, D. and Lapsley H. (1991) *Estimating the Economic Costs of Drug Abuse*, National Campaign Against Drug Abuse, Canberra.

Kickbusch, I. (1988) New perspectives for research in health behaviour, in *Health Behaviour Research and Health Promotion*, (eds R. Anderson *et al.*), Oxford University Press, Oxford, pp. 237–43.

Kickbush, I. (1989) Self-care in health promotion, *Social Science and Medicine*, **29** (2), pp. 125–30.

MacDonald, B. (1974) Evaluation and the control of education, in *Innovation, Evaluation, Research and the Problem of Control*, (eds B. Macdonald and R. Walker), University of East Anglia, Norwich, Norfolk.

Stake, R.E. (1972) An approach to the evaluation of instructional programs: program portrayal vs. analysis, Annual Conference of the American Educational Research Association, Chicago (partially reprinted in *Beyond the Numbers Game*, eds D. Hamilton *et al.*, Macmillan, London, 1977).

Stake, R.E. (1967) The countenance of evaluation, *Teachers' College Record*, **68** (7), pp. 523–40.

CHAPTER 11

Reflexivity: recognizing subjectivity in research

Lynne Stevens

INTRODUCTION

Research in health education is primarily characterized by the use of quantitative methods in which research is performed on and for people. Naturalistic methods which attempt to do research with people are found infrequently in the literature although these methods have often been employed within school settings. This chapter represents the story of my first attempt at doing naturalistic research and is drawn in large part from the methodology section of my Honours thesis in health education which was completed in 1990.

My Honours thesis examined a health education initiative which was launched in a selected group of Victorian primary schools in 1990. The health in primary schools (HIPS) project was developed by Monash University and Victoria College, Burwood, and funded by the Victorian Health Promotion Foundation (VHPF). The VHPF was established by the Victorian State Government under the Tobacco Act (1987) to promote health and prevent disease in Victoria. This act provides for the distribution of funds obtained from a 5% levy on the wholesale price of tobacco products, which netted approximately A$25 million in 1990 (Colquhoun, 1990).

My research was primarily concerned with the implementation of the HIPS project in one school and how top down approaches such as this are mediated and changed in particular contexts.

John Van Maanen (1988) names ethnographic writing that attempts to demystify fieldwork in this way. He offers three basic criticisms of this type of writing, and as this chapter is ostensibly a 'confessional tale' these criticisms should be made explicit here.

First, according to Van Maanen, confessional tales are usually present in a separate methodological section and there is often a clear break between representations of the fieldwork and the actual ethnography. In this way fieldworkers are able to confess to the problems they have experienced in their fieldwork in an abstracted section while largely ignoring these problems when writing the actual ethnography. This could also be a problem inherent in the writing process itself created by the demands of writing a thesis in isolated chapters divorced from each other. Although I do not feel that my work should be criticized on these grounds it is somewhat ironic that what you read here is largely decontextualized as it is only one part of my original thesis.

Second, confessional tales are usually told as a character building tale and are somewhat 'schizophrenic' in nature, oscillating between an 'insider's passionate perspective' and 'an outsider's dispassionate one'. There is usually something of the 'they made me do it' in the writing – limits being characterized as non-negotiable demands imposed on the ethnographer. The third point Van Maanen makes is that these tales are usually presented as a product of mutual understanding. Failures are usually absent.

On the plus side, confessional tales expose the 'interpretive' nature of fieldwork. As Van Maanen says:

> At issue is the fact that there are always many ways to interpret cultural data. Each interpretation can be disputed on many grounds. The data fieldworkers come to hold are not like dollar bills found on the sidewalk and stealthily tucked away in our pockets for later use. Field data are constructed from talk and action (Van Maanen, 1988).

In skilled hands the personal voice can become a self-reflective meditation allowing the reader to gain a deeper sense of the problems posed by the enterprise itself. Van Maanen also views confessional tales as of special interest to students of fieldwork in search of guidance and reassurance. If nothing else I hope this story fulfils that purpose.

ADOPTING A FEMINIST STANDPOINT

Naturalistic research is a tricky business at the best of times. As a novice researcher I found myself negotiating a path characterized by uncertainty and, at times, downright panic. I was unsure what theoretical framework would best suit my intended research and, until quite late in the process, what research question I was endeavouring to answer. My misgivings were only reinforced when I searched through the available literature for a voice that said 'Hey, this is OK, this is how it is', only to find, for the most part, silence. Most research, particularly within health education, was and is written up as a *fait accompli* with very little reference made to the messiness and confusion that I was actually experiencing. What was missing was the researcher's voice. Patti Lather became a bright light that illuminated my way. She focused on reflexive research which as a beginning point recognized the influence of the researcher and emphasized the need to reflect critically on both theory and practice at every moment in the research process.

I had also become increasingly interested in trying to resolve the binary relationship between researcher and researched, a project that I am still pursuing in my PhD research. Research for me has become a 'long conversation' (Silverstone *et al.*, 1984). The word 'conversation' literally means changing together. This chapter represents the beginning of my long conversation.

Liz Stanley and Sue Wise (1990) have listed five related sites that underpin both behaviour and analysis and which for them demonstrate the nature of knowledge in feminist research:

- in the researcher–researched relationship;
- in emotion as a research experience;
- in the intellectual autobiography of the researchers;
- therefore in how to manage the differing 'realities' and understandings of researchers and researched;
- and thus in the complex question of power in research and writing.

Although for me some of these concerns are more important than others at particular times, I try to keep them in mind whenever I try to 'do' research. I remember the internal conflict I experienced at the time I was doing this research. If I was doing feminist research could I then do research with the male teachers and the young boys at the school? Joyce Layland (1990) was also aware of this conflict and had this to say about her research with gay men: 'The latent effect of seeing feminist research as exclusively about women's lives is that it allows things male to go uninvestigated, almost as though the idea of the male-as-norm were not being questioned any more'.

RECOGNIZING SUBJECTIVITY

When using the term 'subjectivity' I borrow from the definition given by Henriques *et al.* (1984) in which they refer to subjectivity as 'individuality and self-awareness'. In referring to subjectivity in this way they do not see 'the subject' of subjectivity as fixed, rather '... subjects are dynamic and multiple, always positioned in relation to particular discourses and practices and produced by these'.

In relation to this Lather (1988) emphasizes that '... ways of knowing are culture-bound and perspectival'. A recognition that we as researchers are ourselves inscribed in dominant discourses in an attempt to avoid the '. . . unhealthy separation between those who know and those who do not' (Scott, 1986.) This recognition may facilitate research that goes some way towards closing the theory/ practice gap.

A focus on subjectivity recognizes '. . . the joint construction of meaning in all social and scientific enquiry' (Roman and Apple, 1990). In according primacy to subjectivity I find it necessary to reject the positivist claim to objectivism which asserts that '. . . knowledge can only be ascribed to that which is founded in "reality" as apprehended by the senses' (Carr and Kemmis, 1986). By viewing knowledge in this way researchers working within the scientific paradigm often render their own cultural beliefs and practices invisible (Roman and Apple, 1990).

In choosing to focus on subjective knowledge I am aware that I could be criticized for treating subjectivity and objectivity as '. . . a binary opposition in which the absence of one implies the presence of the other' (Roman and Apple, 1990). This is not my intention. This view is regarded as too simplistic and denies the interactive relationship between the two. As Roman points out:

> According to this conceptualization, subjectivity is a signpost that distinguishes human consciousness of the social and material world. Its interaction with objectivity is a point of contention in which different but related power struggles take place between and among subordinate and dominant groups over what counts as 'true' knowledge (Roman and Apple, 1990).

Within research into health education the 'scientific' method and emphasis on psychosocial behaviour presupposes some sort of 'essential' subjectivity in which the subject is posited as essentially rational and ultimately predisposed to act in his or her best interests: he or she only remains to be persuaded.

Finding a research topic

When I sat down to write this section of the paper I found my mind drifting, as it often does when I am faced with a worktable full of disordered notes and a mind in approximately the same state. This time however, rather than thinking about anything but the task at hand I found myself reflecting on why and under what circumstances I came to be doing research in health education in the first place.

In the closing stages of a hectic final year of my BA (Ed) I had decided to take up the offer of an Honours year, and had negotiated a supervisor and a topic without fully considering the consequences of my decisions. The fact that I was interested in health education and was given the opportunity to study an innovative programme in this curriculum area was a deciding factor.

At the time I found it difficult to articulate why I was interested in health education. My undergraduate course in education had covered most curriculum areas, many of which I had enjoyed studying, so why health education in particular? During my teaching rounds I had witnessed health education lessons that nearly always used a biomedical discourse that concentrated on imparting facts, was individualistic, and totally abstracted from social context. Having been diagnosed as a diabetic during my adolescence, and having endured countless unsatisfactory encounters with doctors whose only concern was treating the illness and not the social person, perhaps made me sceptical of this approach to health education. The 'critical' approach to health education adopted by my 'soon-to-be' supervisor made explicit the concerns that I had only previously felt implicitly.

Colquhoun (1989) points out that most research students tend to hold a similar paradigmatic stance to their supervisors. At the time I had to make a decision about topic and research orientation, a colleague and myself were in the process of submitting a paper for publication based on a case study we had completed on alcohol education during school rounds the previous year (Colquhoun, Kelly and Stevens, 1990). My supervisor had encouraged us in this pursuit as case studies in primary school health education were few and far between. These circumstances compounded my decision.

Foreshadowed issues

Burgess (1985) notes that while a number of case studies have focused on secondary schools (Hargreaves, 1967; Lacey, 1970; Ball, 1981; Burgess, 1983) there have been few in-depth studies conducted in primary schools . Of those studies that have been completed few have focused specifically on curriculum. The few studies that I am aware of that address the health curriculum (Combes, 1989; Colquhoun, 1989; Beckett, 1990) have focused on the content of curriculum with little attention being given to how this content is mediated through classroom practices.

Previous studies have identified the ideological construct of 'healthism' as the dominant discourse in the health curriculum of primary schools. The regulative discourse (Kirk and Colquhoun (1989) discuss regulative discourse using Bernstein), which promotes the belief that health can be achieved unproblematically through individual effort and discipline, has been variously named as healthism, life-stylism and individualism. These terms are considered to be interchangeable. Healthism is used except where specific authors use one of the other two terms. Healthism works at an ideological level by making it appear natural and given that individuals take responsibility for their own health (Colquhoun, 1990). Cherryholmes suggests that '. . . dominant discourses determine what counts as true, important, relevant and what gets spoken' (McLaren, 1989). It is in this sense that healthism exists as the 'dominant discourse' within health education.

The 'Quit' campaign in Australia (funded by tax revenue on the sale of cigarettes) is a prominent example of articulation of this discourse. This campaign exemplifies what Crawford (1980) terms 'health as self-control' which is characterized by self-denial and self-discipline and sees those individuals who fail to take control of their own health (in this case by giving up smoking) as lacking in willpower or as self-indulgent. The National Campaign Against Drug Abuse (NCADA) uses images of 'fun-loving' young people in its campaigns, for example the 'I'm a w . . . oman' commercial shown on Australian television. This commercial, along with others used in the campaign, places particular emphasis on self-control. However, by promoting images of fun-loving young people, such commercials also present the notion of health as release. The message is that we must exercise self-control and at the same time have fun doing it. Health as self-control denies that people may resort to unhealthy habits in order to find some escape from a world they find less than satisfying. This attitude also denies the socioeconomic and political determinants of smoking.

Naidoo (1986), in critiquing 'individualism' contends that a focus on individual responsiblity for one's own personal behaviour sees a *laissez-faire* attitude adopted by governments because '. . . individual free choice is seen as a desirable goal'. In other words, government intervention is premised on the notion that it is enough for us to have access to knowledge about healthy and unhealthy lifestyle choices. It is then up to us to do something about it. As such, she maintains that coercive measures, such as the legal requirement to wear seat belts, are seen as inappropriate. In this regard it is evident that, in the Australian context at least, we are experiencing an increase in 'coercive' measures, for example, higher taxes on alcohol and cigarettes. However, in the context of primary school health education coercive measures are inappropriate and the voluntaristic or educational model (Tones, 1987) which emphasizes 'informed free choice' is the one most often used. It is in this context that Naidoo's assertions are in evidence.

Three major criticisms against individualistic health education have been formulated by Naidoo (1986):

> . . . first it denies that health is a social product; second, it assumes free choice exists; third, it is not effective within its own terms of reference.

The notion of 'free choice' is considered problematic in a society such as ours which is premised on a hierarchical division of labour, which situates control of the many in the hands of a few and where environmental factors and commercial interests limit free choice (Colquhoun, Kelly and Stevens, 1990).

In effect the notion of free choice is a matter of degree and has a distinct social dimension, factors which are largely ignored by those who adhere to this voluntaristic model. In effect this neglect is a form of social Darwinism where children may come to learn that only the fittest make the healthy choices and survive.

There is ample evidence to suggest that a focus on individual behaviour in order to achieve change in life-style habits has, at best, limited results (Howat and Fisher, 1984). A Health, Education and Welfare Report, *Work in America* (1973), found that diet, exercise, healthcare and heredity predicted only about 25% of the observed mortality from heart disease. The major factor influencing longevity was work satisfaction. With the increasing fiscal crisis and subsequent escalation in the alienation of workers it seems reasonable to assume that the same would apply today. Considering the implications of these findings, which would involve major restructuring of work environments, the emphasis placed on changing individual life-styles is understandable.

One of the main reasons why health prevention measures have failed could be related to the fact that prevention involves convincing people to do something now in order to protect themselves from some future threat to their health. In the case of adolescents in particular, who in many respects see themselves as immortal, this is perhaps an unrealistic expectation. The increasing tendency for governments in Australia to adopt coercive measures to change life-styles is perhaps an indication of the ineffectiveness of the individualistic approach.

It was my original intention to extend this work by documenting instances of healthism in the curriculum at Raneri primary school, which was asked to participate in the pilot phase of the Health in Primary Schools project. (The names of the school and the participants have been changed to achieve anonymity.)

As my fieldwork progressed I became increasingly aware that, although the health curriculum conformed to the pattern I expected, and in many cases its translation into practice served to reinforce the ideological underpinnings of the curricula, instances of resistance to the dominant ideology could be identified. As Cherryholmes points out:

> As soon as you apply a construct it has the effect of emphasizing the sameness of something not the differences ... Constructs and measurements are always interpretations (1988).

By applying the construct of healthism to primary school health education I was in danger of neglecting the exceptions to the rule. I became concerned with explaining why a small minority of teachers resisted (even in small ways) and in turn, given that many teachers had demonstrated that they had a much more comprehensive view of health than was reflected in their teaching, why do they teach health education the way they do? In this regard I found myself focusing on what Hargreaves (1986) terms 'theories of the middle range', i.e. intermediary processes and structures (such as the ethos of the school). As education does not occur in a vacuum it is necessary to link school practices to wider society so that any analysis of schooling needs to be multi-tiered.

Negotiating entry into the school

There were two basic reasons why I chose Raneri primary school for my case study. First, I had been placed at the school for teaching rounds in the last semester of 1989 and had formed the opinion that the staff were a friendly group who would not object to my presence in the school for an extended period. Second, through discussions with my supervising teacher, I had discovered that the school had been chosen as a 'lighthouse school' for the upcoming Health in Primary Schools (HIPS) pilot project, to be initiated in 1990. As such, the project offered me a vehicle for studying two areas of particular interest to me: health education and curriculum innovation.

Dingwall (Burgess, 1985) has referred to a '... hierarchy of consent; a situation in which sponsorship is provided by individuals who stand in positions hierarchically above those who are to be studied'. In this sense my supervisor could be regarded as a sponsor in that his involvement in helping the staff at Raneri to organize the original school submission to the HIPS project obviously influenced the decision to allow me access.

My initial entry into the school was negotiated through a hurried telephone call to the principal on the second to last day of the school year in 1989. I briefly explained my interest in studying the HIPS programme as the basis for my Honours thesis. He was obviously very busy, and after agreeing in principle to my proposal, suggested that I attend an 'in-service' day on aerobics scheduled for the day before school started in 1990.

The in-service day was designed to introduce strategies for teaching aerobics which could be utilized in the exercise component of the programme. My introduction to the assembled teachers as an 'Honours' student from Deakin was accompanied by the light-hearted comment: 'You had better watch what you say and do. She will be writing everything down'. I interpreted this rather unfortunate introduction as evidence that the principal had reservations about my role in the school.

FIELDWORK

The planning

After consultation with my supervisor I decided that I would try and place myself in one classroom in the middle school and one classroom in the upper school in order to gain as wide a perspective of the school as possible given the time constraints I would be forced to work under. Having less than 12 months to complete my study I envisaged that I would have to limit myself to collecting data in the first semester, leaving the second semester in which to collate and complete the analysis of the data, follow up any gaps and write my report. Limiting the scope of the study, whilst at the same time ensuring that I obtained data from as wide a sample as possible, were important considerations.

Negotiating entry to the classrooms for observation proved to be difficult. A protracted industrial dispute over pay and conditions saw teachers adopting a 'work-to-rule' strategy. The principal felt that if I was placed in the classrooms during the dispute participating teachers would be seen to be doing extra work which he felt would be against the spirit of the campaign. In offering this reason for delaying my entry into the school, I am not sure whether he had taken it upon himself to represent the teachers' views or if this strategy had been suggested by the teachers themselves. Given that the principal had demonstrated some reservations about my role, this strategy could simply have been a delaying tactic. His logic, however, demonstrated to me one difference in perceptions of my role as 'participant observer'. My plan was to sit and 'soak up the atmosphere'. I had no intention of increasing the teachers' workload in any way. The principal, however, classified my attendance as 'extra work for the teachers concerned'. On reflection my initial determination to be a 'fly on the wall' was naive. The very act of observation changes the dynamics of classroom interaction.

Walker's comment that case studies represent ' . . . an uncontrolled intervention in the lives of others' (1983) proved to be only too true. The two teachers, knowing they were being observed, set about giving me 'what they thought I wanted' as far as formal health lessons were concerned. The teachers often prefaced their lessons with comments such as 'I hope this lesson provides you with the information you are looking for', and in one particular instance, 'I think you will get something out of this lesson' (Field Notes). In my opinion this resulted in the teachers investing more effort in health lessons than perhaps they would normally have practised, given the evidence obtained in interviews which showed that health lessons were, for the most part, treated incidentally and conducted infrequently. This situation indicates the importance of multiple data gathering strategies.

I was also unaware until much later on in the life of this project that the teachers received the impression from the principal that I would be visiting their classroom for only one day. This amounted to a major misunderstanding of my intentions on the principal's part and could go some way towards explaining the difficulties I faced in the grade 5/6 classroom during the period I was conducting fieldwork. Burgess (1985) documents the process of renegotiation with teachers who were not fully aware of her intentions during her case study. It seems that misconceptions about researchers' intentions are a common problem with this type of research.

The practise

My fieldwork consisted of taking detailed notes on informal teacher/pupil/researcher interaction, activities related to the Recreation, Exercise and Diet programme (RED), health lessons and indeed all other lessons conducted over the course of one day in the selected grades. Acting on my supervisor's instructions to be a 'sponge', I initially took down every word that passed the teachers' and students' lips. This proved to be completely exhausting and, considering the amount of paper I used in the process, environmentally irresponsible. However, this strategy did prove useful in identifying the types of interaction that existed in each classroom and indeed across different curriculum areas in the one classroom. This strategy also helped me identify emerging issues, enabling me to effectively narrow my focus as time went on. For example, it became evident that the teacher in one classroom employed a different pedagogical approach when teaching health as compared with mathematics. This led me to consider the hidden messages she conveyed to pupils about the status of subjects with important implications for teaching health.

Burgess (1985) decided not to make diary entries during the lessons she was observing because she considered this would be too threatening, instead she relied on her memory to write up observations after the classes. Sue McGrath (Grade 3/4 teacher) commented on one occasion that she wondered why I wrote down every word she said. On other occasions my note taking did not seem to affect her. Although I was aware that my actions could be threatening, I did not trust myself to remember what transpired in the course of the school day and opted to take detailed notes.

In spite of my prolific supply of raw data, however, I am acutely aware that case studies suffer from being only partial accounts of any given situation, '. . . it [the case study] captures an instant in time and space that can then be held against a moving changing reality' (Walker, 1983).

The people

During the course of my research I interviewed the principal, deputy principal, all available staff, eight children from grade 3/4, and four children from grade 5/6, together with my supervisor who played an active part in the HIPS programme as an official evaluator at another primary school.

My two 'key informants' for this study were in effect chosen by the principal who acted as the 'gatekeeper' for my research (Burgess, 1985). The principal decided when I was to gain access to the classroom and which teachers would be the most suitable for my research purposes. Given the authority relationships within the school and between myself (as a junior researcher) and the principal there seemed to be no other alternative.

Gold (1958, cited in Burgess, 1985) suggests four major roles for collecting data by 'participant observation': the complete participant, the complete observer, the participant as observer and the observer as participant. Pryce (1979, cited in Burgess, 1985) maintains:

> What the interviewer is influences and maybe determines the kind of data he or she receives. There are a number of factors; age, gender, and ethnicity are probably the most significant.

I consider that it was no accident that in the Grade 3/4 classroom with a female teacher I was assigned the role of observer as participant, whilst in the Grade 5/6 classroom with a male teacher I was never allowed to be more than an observer. My only participation involved photocopying extra sheets when the teacher miscalculated the number required for the lesson in progress.

Although both classrooms could be considered to be 'information rich' (indeed any classroom would be if you looked long and hard enough), the grade 3/4 teacher proved to be a researcher's dream come true. She was co-operative, interested, and friendly. From the outset I was considered to be part of the furniture, called on to help with reading and to participate in classroom activities and excursions. The grade 5/6 teacher however, whilst maintaining a veneer of friendship and co-operation demonstrated resistance to my presence in his classroom. This resistance manifested itself in various ways. On several occasions he simply 'forgot' that I was coming into the class to observe that day and as a result had not planned a health lesson.

When it came to interview times, three separate appointments were made with this teacher. None were kept. On two occasions meetings over-ran into appointment times and on one occasion an all day excursion had been planned which he simply forgot to tell me about.

Walker (1983) posed the question:

> How does [the researcher] avoid the danger of over-involvement with certain groups with the possible consequence of over-representing their perspective in his [sic] eventual report?

My response to this question would be that it is almost impossible to do so. What needs to be done, however, is to acknowledge this over-involvement and to find ways of using it to lead to a better understanding of the particular social milieu that any researcher will find themselves involved in. McRobbie (1982) sounded a warning to ethnographers who wish to disguise the '. . . economic, cultural and political conditions under which they labour'. She went on to note:

> . . . ethnographers' retelling of their fieldwork often mystifies or obscures the complexities and messiness of situating one's own interests and experiences when analysing data from interviews and participant observation (McRobbie, 1982).

Indeed, if I was to attempt to present a dematerialized account of my research and cut out the 'messiness' I would rob myself and the reader of a precious vehicle for understanding the different pedagogies that existed and how they manifested themselves in the different approaches to health education that were evident in the school.

It is a fact of life that it is relatively easy to develop a rapport with some people whilst with others it becomes a continual struggle to reach some sort of common ground. I firmly believe that my somewhat dubious status as a student researcher, and a female one at that, affected the relationships I had with both the male and older female staff members at the school. Ultimately what this meant for my research was a personal struggle in which I endeavoured to account for the different personalities I encountered only as they related to my research interests. I do not make the claim that I was always successful.

Scott (1986) talked about the differential relationships between herself and the people she interviewed. She documented how she gained immediate rapport with the women she interviewed who were, admittedly, of a similar age and enjoyed a similar status within the academic community she was investigating. The same was not true of the men she interviewed:

> I found the same level of rapport impossible to achieve in most cases. Now, I do not want to suggest that we had any real difficulty in gaining and carrying out interviews with men . . . what we did find . . . was a difference in the form and quality of many of the interviews with men (1986).

I also found this to be the case with the men I interviewed. Both the principal and the deputy principal at Raneri asserted their authority by putting strict limits on the time available for interviews indicating that they were extremely busy. Peter Farnsworth, another male teacher at the school, continually made comments such as 'Oh, not you again' and 'Why do you need to collect so much data? Anyone would think you were doing a PhD'. These comments were made when I passed him in the corridor or when we met in the staff room. In a later interview with him he presented as very offhand and flippant. For example, when I tried to elicit responses from him regarding the teaching of wider social issues in health education, the following was a typical response:

Lynne: What about the link between health education and environmental education? To me that seems like a chance to get the kids to look at wider social issues and try and do something about things that ...

Peter: Things like poverty? What are we going to do about that?

Lynne: That was an example ...

Peter: Oh, was it? (laughter) It was a good one.

Not all interviews with male staff members were this difficult. The point to be made here is that, unlike the women I interviewed, generally the men were at pains to demonstrate that they were in control of the interview situation. I should also point out that some of the older women at Raneri were extremely reluctant to be interviewed. After considerable negotiation several agreed to be interviewed at 3 p.m. when they knew the interview would be limited to half an hour. One teacher, Anne Murphy, spent the whole interview shuffling papers around on her desk and looking at the clock.

The different perceptions of the purpose of my research demonstrated by individual teachers concretely affected the 'tone' of my interviews and subsequently the data I was able to collect from them.

The lack of enthusiasm demonstrated by some teachers was, I feel, due in no small measure to the difficulty in relating esoteric theories to the everyday world of the teachers couched in language that was intelligible to them. This is not meant to imply any lack of sophistication on the part of the teachers I encountered. It is more a criticism of the language that is used in such discourses, which very often presupposes considerable *a priori* knowledge of the theoretical constructs used by researchers.

As an example, the grade 5/6 teacher I observed asked me at least three times in as many weeks what the purpose of my research was. To be fair I would have to say that on reflection I probably gave him three different versions. Taking a grounded theory approach may well be a device that enables you to rework ideas in the light of emerging data, but, as Glaser notes:

> ... generating theory is done by a human being who at times is intimately involved with and other times quite distant from data – and who is surely plagued by other conditions in his life (cited in Sparkes, 1986).

The 'other conditions' may well have been my feelings of being an intruder in this particular classroom which made me loath to make known my uncertainties about the direction of my research for fear of losing what little credibility I had gained. In the more supportive atmosphere of the grade 3/4 classroom I felt less threatened and therefore I was able to give active voice to my emerging theories and accompanying confusion.

Interviews

I approach the subject of interviews with some trepidation as this aspect of my research proved the most problematic from a methodological, practical, and personal viewpoint.

The setting

All interviews were recorded on a small hand-held recorder. I decided on this strategy so that I could concentrate on the meaning of what was being said rather than concentrating on the mechanical aspect of recording all the words by hand. None of the teachers objected to this method, although some were more nervous than others and made comments such as 'I sound dreadful on tape'. Before commencing the interviews, I made sure that interviewees were aware that their anonymity would be preserved and that they would be the only ones who had access to the transcripts other than myself. The interviews with teachers were conducted for the most part during their time release and in their individual classrooms. This required perseverance on my part and a great deal of co-operation by the teachers. Staff meetings and unplanned interruptions caused constant revision of interview times. One teacher whose programme was changed at the last minute accommodated me by suggesting we talk in the corridor whilst her grade 2 class worked largely unattended. This proved to be quite disastrous as the children kept interrupting to tell tales or to ask for directions. The noise level almost amounted to noise pollution and made transcription of this interview particularly arduous.

Cole (1984) recognizing the constraints placed on teachers when interviewed in the classroom situation (especially when asked to comment on sensitive issues), interviewed teachers in his study away from the institutional setting. This seems to be a reasonable strategy. However, given my own personal time constraints together with my wish not to impose on teachers unduly, I felt that this was not an option open to me. Cole qualifies his interview strategy by recognizing that teachers still may present themselves in certain strategic ways despite the interview setting.

Theoretical saturation

Judging how much data was 'enough' was a real problem for me. Even now I am concerned that I failed to interview two staff members whom I found it impossible to catch up with, although I am aware that I did reach the point of theoretical saturation long before I stopped interviewing. (Agar [1980] uses this term to describe the point when the data becomes repetitive.) Scott summed up the problem when reflecting on her own interviewing experiences:

> We developed a tendency to press on with the interviewing in the belief that this in itself was the most important part of the research even when we were already 'saturated' with data. We had fallen into the positivistic trap even though methodologically we thought we had located ourselves outside that framework. We were treating ourselves simply as receptacles for the experiences of others and often ignored as data our own experiences of the process (1986).

The questions

Interviews were largely unstructured with the intention of avoiding the imposition of the interviewer's prior conceptual framework (Cole, 1984), although I am now aware that '... what we want to collect data **for** decides what data we collect' (Lather, 1988). As Agar points out:

> You do not go into the field as a passive recorder of objective data – as you choose what to attend to and how to interpret it, mental doors slam shut on the alternatives (1980).

As well as being aware that my own prior conceptual framework affected what I attended to in interviews it soon became evident that my previous introduction to the staff had given them certain preconceptions regarding the purpose of my interviews (see p. 159). I also found it difficult initially to avoid posing leading questions. In an attempt to overcome these methodological constraints I allowed the interviewees to expound as much as they liked on any one subject in the hope of negating these influences. I believe that this strategy was largely successful. However, it did leave me with an overwhelming amount of interview data to transcribe and analyse.

What should I transcribe?

In condensing the interviews into a case study researchers can commit all kinds of 'methodological violence' on data which is difficult for subjects to control (Walker, 1983).

The process of transcribing my interviews led me to a lot of soul searching. Should I synthesize the interview data so that it presented the views of the interviewees in spirit rather than in form thereby cutting down on transcription time? Or should I report the interviews word for word? I had a 'gut' feeling that to synthesize the interviews, thus relying on my interpretation of what should or should not be regarded as important, was somehow an unwarranted intrusion on the meanings of those that I had interviewed. After all, my interpretations would need to be called into play yet again when it came time to decide what to include in the final thesis. The problems inherent in selecting data for the final report were exemplified by Burgess when she noted:

Indeed a major problem overall proved to be the selection of material on the basis of particular themes for inclusion in the final report. In the process of this selection a wealth of data which had been collected was left undisturbed and unaccounted for (1985).

SUMMARY

The selection of an appropriate research methodology and the need to subsequently justify that selection can be likened to jumping from an aeroplane and discovering that your parachute will not open. Nothing is certain, everything is problematic. You resolve one dilemma only to have it replaced by several more. Questions regarding subjectivity, ownership of data, how to obtain data without compromising the people being researched, how to remain objective enough to distinguish between people's reasoned objections and false consciousness, how to decide if in fact it is not you that is suffering from 'ideological block'; all remain largely unanswered. In the end the best way perhaps is to learn by your mistakes. As Lather so aptly states:

The new historians of science have made it clear that methodological questions are decided in the practice of research by those committed to developing the best possible answers to their questions, not by armchair philosophers of research. Let us get on with the task (1983).

ENDNOTE

As a final comment I would like to include the endnote in my original thesis. Although it is presented in a decontextualized form it serves as a representation of the transient quality of any naturalistic research which, when presented in written form, represents a 'frozen' moment in time. I am acutely aware that those people involved in the project in an ongoing capacity may already have worked towards resolving some of the issues identified in the main body of my thesis. In this regard I leave the reader with these final words:

> I have reached no conclusions, have created no boundaries.
> shutting out and shutting in separating inside
>   from outside: I have
>   drawn no line;
>   as
>   manifold events of sand
>   change the dune's shape that will not be the same
>   shape
>   tomorrow,
>   so I am willing to go along, to accept
>   the becoming
>   thought, to stake off no beginnings or ends,
>   to establish
> no walls . . .
>   (Ammons, 1977).

REFERENCES

Agar, M. (1980) *The Professional Stranger: An Informal Introduction to Ethnography*, Academic Press, New York.

Ammons, A.R. (1977) Corson's Inlet, *The Selected Poems*, pp. 43–4, New York.

Ball, S.J. (1981) *Beachside Comprehensive: A Case Study of Secondary Schooling*, Cambridge University Press, Cambridge.

Beckett, L. (1990) A critical edge to school health education, *Unicorn*, **16** (2), pp. 90–99.

Burgess, H. (1985) Case Study and Curriculum Research: Some Issues for Teacher Researchers, in Burgess, R.G., *Issues in Educational Research: Qualitative Methods*, The Falmer Press, London, pp. 177–92.

Burgess, R.G. (1983) *Experiencing Comprehensive Education: A Study of Bishop McGregor School*, Methuen, London.

Burgess, R.G. (1985) *Strategies in Educational Research*, The Falmer Press, London.

Carr, W. and Kemmis, S. (1986) *Becoming Critical: Knowing Through Action Research*, Deakin University Press, Geelong.

Cherryholmes, C.H. (1988) Construct Validity and the Discourses of Research, *American Journal of Education*, **96** (3), pp. 421–57.

Cole, M. (1984) Teaching till two thousand: teachers' consciousness in times of crisis, in *Social Crisis and Educational Research* (eds L. Barton & S. Walker) Croom Helm, Canberra.

Colquhoun, D. (1990) *Health Based Physical Education and the Health in Primary Schools Project*, paper presented to the AISEP Conference, Loughborough, England.

Colquhoun, D., Kelly, P. and Stevens, L. (1990) Individualism in School Health Education: A Case Study of Alcohol Education in a Victoria Primary School, *Achper National Journal*, **128**, pp. 6–8.

Colquhoun, L. (1989) *Healthism and Health Based Physical Ecducation: A Critique*, unpublished PhD thesis, University of Queensland.

Coombes, G. (1989) The ideology of health education in schools, *British Journal of Sociology of Education*, **10** (1).

Crawford, R. (1980) Healthism and the medicalization of everyday life, *International Journal of Health Services*, **10** (3), pp. 365–89.

Gold, R. (1958) Roles in sociological field observation, *Social Forces*, **36** (3), pp. 217–33.

Hammersley, M. and Atkinson, P. (1983) *Ethnography: Principles in Practice*, Tavistock Publications, London and New York.

Hargreaves, D.H. (1967) *Social Relations in a Secondary School*, Routledge and Kegan Paul, London.

Hargreaves, J. (1986) *Sport, Power and Culture: A Social and Historical Analysis of Popular Sports in Britain*, Polity Press, Cambridge.

Henriques, J., Hollway, W., Urwin, C., Venn, C., and Walkerdine, V. (1984) *Changing the Subject*, Methuen, London and New York.

Howat, P. and Fisher, J. (1984) Health education for self-responsibility or health education for structural perspectives? *Achper National Journal*, **104**, pp. 5–9.

Kirk, D. and Colquhoun, D. (1989) Healthism and physical education, *British Journal of Sociology of Education*, **10** (4), pp. 417–34.

Lacey, C. (1970) *Hightown Grammar: The school as a Social System*, Manchester University Press, Manchester.

Lather, P. (1988) Feminist Perspectives on Empowering Research Methodologies, in *Women's Studies Int. Forum*, **11** (6), pp. 569–81.

Lather, P. (1989) Deconstructing/deconstructive Enquiry: The Politics of Knowing and Being Known, paper presented at the American Educational Research Association Annual Conference, San Francisco, California.

Lather, P. (1983) Research as Praxis, *Harvard Educational Review*, **56** (3), pp. 257–73.

McLaren, P. (1989) *Life in Schools: An Introduction to Critical Pedagogy in the Foundations of Education*, Longman, New York & London.

McRobbie, A. (1982) The Politics of Feminist Research: Between Text, Talk and Action, *Feminist Review*, pp. 46–57.

Measor, L. (1985) Interviewing: A Strategy in Qualitative Research, in *Strategies of Educational Research*, (ed. R.G. Burgess), The Falmer Press, pp. 55–77.

Naidoo, J. (1986) Limits to Individualism, in *The Politics of Health Education: Raising the Issues* (eds S. Rodmell and A. Watt), Routledge and Kegan Paul, London, pp. 17–37.

Roman, L. and Apple, M. (1990) Is Naturalism a Move Away From Positivism? Materialist and Feminist Approaches to Subjectivity in Ethnographic Research, in *Qualitative Enquiry in Education*, (eds E. Eisner and A. Peshkin), Teacher's College Press, New York, pp. 1–44.

Scott, S. (1986) Feminist Research and Qualitative Methods: A Discussion of Some of the Issues, in *Issues in Educational Research: Qualitative Methods* (ed. G. Burgess), The Falmer Press, London, pp. 67–88.

Silverstone, R., Hirsch, E. and Morley, D. (1991) Listening to a long conversation: an ethnographic approach to the study of information and communication technologies in the home, *Curriculum Studies*, 5 (2), pp. 204–27.

Sparkes, A.C. (1986) Beyond description: The Need for Theory Generation in Physical Education, *Physical Education Review*, 9 (1), pp. 41–9.

Stanley, L. (ed) (1990) *Feminist Praxis: Research, Theory, and Epistemology in Feminist Sociology*, Routledge.

Tones, K. (1987) Health promotion, effective education and personal-social development, in *Health Education in Schools* (eds K. David and T. Williams), Harper & Row, London.

Van Maanen, J. (1988) *Tales of the Field: On Writing Ethnography*, The University of Chicago Press, Chicago, Ill.

Walker, R. (1980) The Conduct of Educational Case Studies: Ethics, Theory and Procedures, in *Rethinking Educational Research* (eds W.B. Docksell and D. Hamilton), Hodder & Stoughton, London, pp. 30–63.

Walker, R. (1983) Three good reasons for not doing case studies in curriculum research, *Curriculum Studies Journal*, 15 (2), pp. 155–165.

CHAPTER 12

Researching women's health

Liz Eckermann

POLITICAL BACKGROUND

In his foreword to an issues paper on Researching Women's Health for the Australian Commonwealth Department of Health, Housing and Community Services, Brian Howe, Minister for that department, argued that 'the principles set out in the National Women's Health Policy are sound', and he claimed that he is 'confident that research undertaken in line with (the Policy's recommendations) ... will significantly increase our understanding of the social and environmental factors which affect women's health' (Kane, 1991).

In the same year (1991) a senior official of the Australian Commonwealth Department of Health, Housing and Community Services 'challenged the legality of the Federal Government's women's health programme in the Federal Court and accused a sex discrimination commissioner of bias against men' (Kingston, 1991).

These two anomalous positions on the legitimacy of 'women only' health services and policy from within the Commonwealth Department may seem a trivial matter. Many perceived the challenge to 'women only' services as a joke which would fade in time. The issue has not faded. The challenge continues and gains momentum as the case moves to the Human Rights and Equal Opportunities Commission. The existence of 'women only' health services in Australia was under serious threat in 1992 and with it the legitimacy of research on women's health.

HISTORY

Wass (1992) traces the history of the Women's Health Movement in Australia to the 1970s. The movement grew out of an amalgamation of the wider women's movement and the 'social health'

movement of the WHO. By the 1980s, Wass argues, many state governments and the Federal Health Department had started to recognize
that health was a social justice issue. The Women's Movement and
the New Public Health Movement came together under a social justice
banner. There were also parallels which developed between consumer
groups, professional groups (especially with the professionalization
of nurses and social workers), women's interest groups and various
pressure groups.

The process of gathering support for the Women's Health Movement culminated in the National Women's Health Policy launched
by the then Australian Prime Minister, Bob Hawke, in April 1989.

The policy report recognized the need for affirmative action in the
area of women's health and put forward recommendations for priority
action in five areas including 'research and data collection on women's
health' (Kane, 1991).

Based on interviews and consultations with over a million women,
the report prioritized seven health issues for improving the health
of Australian women. They are: 'reproductive health and sexuality;
the health of ageing women; women's emotional and mental health;
violence against women; occupational health and safety; the health
needs of carers; and the health effects of sex role stereotyping'
(Commonwealth Department Community Services and Health,
1989). In a 1991 response to the recommendations of the report,
Howe (Minister of the Department concerned) argued that he was
'particularly concerned that Australia's major research funding
bodies and tertiary institutions undertaking medical research should
address issues (of priority in women's health)', and went on to
suggest that improving women's health would have a multiplier
effect since:

> The development of more appropriate intervention strategies will
> not only improve the health of Australian women but have an
> effect on the well-being of all Australians for, as in the words
> of Dr Hiroshi Nakajima, Director General of the World Health
> Organization 'Women are the key to achieving health for all'
> (Kane, 1991).

The future of research in women's health thus seemed assured,
not only on affirmative action grounds but also on classical liberal 'common good' grounds. However, the challenge in the Federal Court and
in the Human Rights and Equal Opportunities Commission, has sent
researchers, service providers and policy makers in women's health
back to their bunkers. The need seems to have arisen yet again to
defend research into women's health. The basic questions of 'Why
do we need "women only" health research?' and 'What is it that is
unique about this area that requires specific attention?' are being asked

again. We need to develop creative and unequivocal responses to such questions.

The anti-women only services case is based on three major objections – one legalistic and 'moral', one empirical and the other political. The legalistic arm of the challenge rests within an interpretation of equal opportunity legislation – both the spirit and the letter of such legislation. The empirical strand of the challenge is based on using mortality rates as the ultimate indicator of the health status of a population. The argument is put forward that since Australian males have a life expectancy at birth of 5–8 years less than that of Australian females (Australian Institute of Health, 1990) males are in greater need of additional or 'special' services and research. Morbidity rates, which are much higher among Australian women than Australian men (Australian Institute of Health, 1990) are ignored as a key health indicator. Specifically, in this case the compression of morbidity as the population ages is ignored as a major health issue affecting more aged women than men. Similarly the extent to which social, economic and occupational deprivation can act as social indicators of health status in women is ignored. Angie Smith (1992) argues that if we are to fully explore social aspects of health, including the power that women can summon as consumers of health, we need to ask questions such as 'Who has the knowledge? Who has the power? Who has the money?' given that 'education, politics and wealth' may be key indicators of 'the relative status of the sexes' (Smith, 1992).

This leads us to the third strand of the anti-women only services debate – the political argument about sectional competition for resources. Arndt (1992) argues that the anti-women only lobby was less concerned with 'exploring men's specific health requirements and catering to those needs' than with 'politically motivated groups who hijack community resources for their section interests' (Arndt, 1992). If women only health services are detracting from funding for aged care, Aboriginal health, the poor, men and other interest groups, those supporting the anti-women's health services argument have not been able to show any evidence to support their case.

Wass (1992) takes the political argument one step further, arguing that even the new legitimacy of women's health issues which followed on from the National Women's Health Policy statements should be viewed with some suspicion. She argues that 'while these developments may have sprung from politicians with the best of intentions, the manner in which they are being implemented may do more to exploit women than empower them', a phenomenon which 'does not necessarily augur well for the Women's Health Movement' (Wass, 1992). Examples of where the 'process' of implementing women's health policy has gone against the tenets of participation have been mammography screening and osteoporosis prevention (Short, 1992; Wass, 1992).

WHY WOMEN'S HEALTH?

Within the political climate outlined above we need to mount creative and imaginative responses to answer the question 'Why women's health'? To achieve this we need to examine theoretical, methodological, political, economic and ethical issues which relate to women's health research.

Given the complex relationship between health status and the social, political, economic and physical environment which is well documented in the literature (Brown, 1976; SAHC, 1990; Gardner, 1992; Lupton and Najman, 1989; Davis and George, 198; Bates and Linder-Pelz, 1990; Palmer and Short, 1989), it would seem essential to start with a social model of health to fully encapsulate the health concerns of women. In fact some authors argue that the 'medical model' is anathema to women's health given that 'an emphasis on women's health, as opposed to the diagnosis and treatment of women's illness, already implies a rejection of the traditional (patriarchal) medical model' (McBride and McBride, 1981).

A social model would seem to lend itself to sociological analysis. However, the dilemma for sociologists attempting to understand women's health issues is that the classical theoretical tradition in sociology is essentially 'masculine' and 'disembodied'.

THEORETICAL ISSUES

The classical tradition in sociology like the historical tradition of Western thought generally 'has been hostile to women' (McBride and McBride, 1981). It is thus no wonder that it has little to say about women, let alone women's health. No attempt is made in classical sociology to deconstruct patriarchal social relations. Despite some attempts to defend Marx, Weber, Durkheim and Simmel as having dealt with 'the woman question' (Kandal, 1988) most writers agree that women are notably absent from sociology's classical tradition (Stacey and Thorne, 1985; McBride and McBride, 1981).

The sociological theorists of the early to mid 20th century offer little more. Parsons (1951) in discussing the 'sick role' pays little attention to women's health. In characterizing women as being involved with 'affective' characteristics in the family his arguments merely reinforce existing patriarchal relations. Parsons' expanded psychodynamic model of the 'sick role', which identifies illness as motivated deviance, explicitly refers only to males (Parsons, 1964).

The tradition which does address the specific concerns of women and does offer a sociology of the body is phenomenology. The popularity of the phenomenological tradition in current research on women's health underscores the extent to which 'women's health at the core means taking women's lived experience as the starting point for all health efforts'. (McBride and McBride, 1981). McBride and McBride argue that women's health research has started to bring '"lived experience" to a place . . . of honour within the dominant . . . conceptual frameworks of Western society' and that such an emphasis has philosophical ethical and 'methodological consequences' (McBride and McBride, 1981).

Not only are there distinctions **between** women in relation to age, class, ethnicity, geographical location, sexual preference and political beliefs but also **within** individual women there may be multiple realities. In post-industrial Western societies women are typically multiply constituted as worker, housekeeper and mother. McBride and McBride extend the argument to suggest that women 'exist in a context that may be constantly in flux' such that 'no single point of view about women's health can ever be expected to emerge'. They suggest that it is inappropriate to 'differentiate women as a group', rather, we 'have to analyse the experiences of individual women' because to generalize beyond the population under scrutiny in research endeavours 'may be destructive to an appreciation of others' lived experiences' (McBride and McBride, 1981). The implication is that we need to adopt unique theoretical frameworks, with unique methodological implications, to tap into the specific lived experiences of individual women if we are to gain a clear understanding of women's health issues.

METHODOLOGICAL ISSUES

Bryman (1984) argues that there is 'no clear symmetry between epistemological positions (e.g. phenomenology, positivism) and associated techniques of social research (e.g. participant observation, social survey)' (Bryman, 1984). However, he does argue for an epistemological hiatus between the 'methodologies' (as opposed to 'methods') of quantitative and qualitative research.

The question arises as to whether an intellectual commitment to a philosophical position directly determines the methods of research at the researcher's disposal (Lofland, 1976). Does a commitment to a feminist philosophical viewpoint mean that only a limited range of research methods are available to the researcher in examining women's health?

Some writers on research methods argue that technical issues decide the appropriate method to be used. Trow (1957) argued for 'the problem under investigation properly dictating the methods of investigation' (cited in Bryman, 1984). Bryman (1984) suggested that an epistemological premise may determine the way the problem is posed, but once defined the problem could be explained via any technique.

I would suggest the need to go even further than Trow and Bryman in deconstructing the orthodox view of dichotomous (quantitative and qualitative) research traditions. A plethora of factors influences the research process, not the least of which is the context in which the research occurs. Bryman and Trow tend to assume an ideal type 'vacuum' for the research process, untainted by such mundane matters as the views of funding agencies. There appears to be a need to add political, economic and social factors as significant variables in determining both the way the research problem is posed and the techniques used to generate data. Issues such as convention, the potential use of the research, the perceived audience for the research and funding bodies' views on 'legitimate' research endeavours all significantly influence the research process. This has been particularly relevant in women's health research in reference to submissions for funding by the Australian National Health and Medical Research Council (NH and MRC), the Australian Research Council (ARC), and the Research and Development Grants Advising Committee (RADGAC).

Between 1985 and 1989 the Medical Research Committee of the NH and MRC funded 92 women's health projects (2.4% of the total of funded projects) and 'the Public Health and Research Development Committee supported – nine' (13.6% of the total). 'RADGAC allocated ... 9.1% of its funding between 1984 and 1988 to seven projects concerned with women's health issues' (Kane, 1991). The low levels of funding partly reflected lower submission rates from researchers on women's health but also higher rejection rates of research proposals.

Bryman notes that 'few researchers traverse the epistemological hiatus which opens up between the research traditions' (Bryman, 1984). Where attempts have been made to combine qualitative and quantitative approaches, qualitative research is often seen as exploratory preparation (or 'foreplay') for quantitative research ('the real thing'). It is often seen as 'occupying a lower rung on the epistemological ladder' or 'representing the fodder for quantitative researchers'. Thus the assumed polarity remains, with qualitative analysis being considered 'soft, subjective and speculative', while quantitative analysis is described as 'hard, objective and rigorous' (Bryman, 1984) – or in more gynocentric language 'wet' and 'dry' analysis (Roberts, 1981).

The costs of following the qualitative road are problems of legitimacy especially in approaching research funding bodies. One response is to question the criteria of legitimacy currently used by many research funding bodies and professional journals and to promote arguments about the validity of qualitative research findings. Phenomenology, post-structuralism and post-modernism all provide theoretical launching pads to mount an attack on scientism, positivism and the Western rational tradition.

Another path is to accept the primacy of subjective experience as the appropriate expression of women's experience of their health but to acknowledge that any issue also has a politico-economic and a broader social context. Thus one can be eclectic, without betraying a feminist stance on research by acknowledging that at different levels of analysis different theoretical and methodological frameworks are appropriate. Like Turner (1987) I would argue that using phenomenological theory and interviewing techniques to tap the subjective experience of women talking about their health does not preclude using other theoretical, methodological and technical frameworks at the politico-economic and social levels. With Furler (1985) and Kane (1991) I would emphasize the need to 'improve the national health data base' on women's health and to expand 'epidemiological research which enquires into patterns of morbidity and mortality accompanying the reality of women's lives in a partriarchal and capitalist society' (Furler, 1985).

In 1993, the Australian Bureau of Statistics will release a National Women's Publication which will go some way towards satisfying that wish list. The National Women's Publication will address the social position of women and provide data which will allow researchers to draw connections between social position and health status.

Although such 'positivistically' collected data does not accord with the feminist principles of tapping into women's lived experience, it does provide information that can be used to further the cause of women. As Dorothy Broom (1991) argues:

The feminist analysis of health and illness emphasizes the importance of women's social position in the production of their ill health. This understanding, more recently labelled the 'social views of health' underlies the two aims of the women's health movement: to change the overall social structure which is sickening to women, while at the same time providing improved individual services, health information and health education to women whose personal health is compromised.

To achieve these aims we need both qualitative and quantitative data. We need to know how many women are affected by particular health problems. We need to be able to name eating disorders, depression or repetitive strain injury as major public health problems requiring a major injection of resources for research, services and policy. Unless the appropriate epidemiological research is carried out we cannot give individuals suffering from these problems a voice. Alongside the macro-picture we can place the 'full, contextually-rich descriptions (of the) first-person experiences of women' which can also significantly influence policy (McBride and McBride, 1981).

A CASE STUDY: RESEARCHING EATING 'DISORDERS'

One way that women have been able to project a 'voice' in protest against a patriarchal world is to use their bodies as a script of disquiet. Anorexia nervosa and bulimia can be seen as two such scripts.

Many conventional research accounts of eating disorders identify such phenomena as a problem from the perspective of all involved, including the person with the 'disorder', and offer aetiological explanations to further treatment, prevention and policy. Few researchers ask the subjects of their research whether they perceive their behaviour as a problem, and even if such a question is asked, the answer is not taken seriously. The normalizing gaze of the researcher, the medical profession, and especially the psychiatric profession, renders the 'problem' as given and in need of being rectified.

It was with that evangelical spirit that I entered the fray on eating disorders research. Having experienced several people close to me developing anorexia nervosa and having worked as a telephone counsellor and consultant for an eating disorders self-help group, I felt I had the necessary close-hand experience to truly understand the phenomenon. I set forth to explain eating disorders from a sociological perspective with the aim of putting in place prevention programmes to rid the world forever of the scourge of eating disorders. My training as an academic sociologist influenced the way I posed the problem, the aetiological factors that I sought out and my prescriptions for change. The fact that I am a woman led me to believe that I had privileged access to the world of eating disorders, which is largely inhabited by women. However, fairly early in my research endeavours I was dealt several conceptual blows by the people whom I was researching.

The first problem was dealing with the terminology. Should I accept the diagnostic categories of the psychiatric profession or should I find an alternative way of expressing the phenomena encapsulated within the Diagnostic Statistical Manual III and IIIR (American Psychiatric Association) categories of anorexia nervosa and bulimia? If such 'disorders' are socially constructed, was the most appropriate task to deconstruct such notions and leave the health policy implications aside? This seems to be a problem faced by many social researchers in the health field who are trying to escape the deterministic implications of a medical model of the health issue which they are addressing. How do you talk about health issues outside of medical terminology? Is it possible to 'bracket' (Husserl, 1952) assumptions about reality? Following a strict social constructionist path tends to create more problems than it solves, especially when it regresses to a social constructionist view of the human body. The path which I found most comfortable was to accept that the psychiatric categories anorexia nervosa and bulimia are socially constructed and in need of deconstruction but that the body has some ontological reality in biology. It is the way that the body is presented and represented in time and space that is open to question rather than its ontological existence. I chose to continue using a qualified sense of the labels anorexia nervosa and bulimia (despite both being serious misnomers for the lived experience of women) because to locate the behaviours as a serious public health issue I was obliged to use epidemiological research which had been based on the diagnostic categories. This is not to say that over time other ways of characterizing similar behaviour may not be developed and that these new characterizations may be able to tap into the 'public issue' dimension of women's private troubles. This stance may be seen as representing rampant pragmatism or crass expediency but it was the only way that I knew how to use the sociological imagination in converting private troubles to public issues.

My next setback was making an oversocialized assumption about my interviewees. Like Orbach (1985) I had assumed that the mass media was a key to understanding anorexia nervosa. I presumed that the messages contained in the 'mass of media persuasion which stresses the necessity of slimness to a woman's survival' had 'become insinuated into each woman's experience of self and (found) their expression in each woman's relationship to her body' (Orbach, 1985). One of the dimensions of difference between people who develop anorexia and those who do not, appeared to be encapsulated in the notion that 'the anorexic woman has absorbed from early on more intensely, the very same messages that all girls receive' (Orbach, 1985).

The young women I was researching disagreed. They found it arrogant and offensive that I should assume a hypodermic thesis of media effects on 'impressionable' young minds. What evidence did I have, they asked, that they were more susceptible to media messages than the rest of the population. On reflection, I realized that I had privileged the structural side of the structure/agency dimension. Allowing my interviewees a strong sense of individual agency, by taking seriously their representations of their anorexia or bulimia in the unstructured interviews, enabled me to reconceptualize anorexia and bulimia as 'solutions' rather than 'problems' from my interviewees' points of view.

A similar misunderstanding between my own and my interviewees' perceptions arose in relation to the role of the family in generating eating disorders. I came to the conclusion that invoking the family and the mass media as scapegoats for the current epidemic of eating 'disorders', although sociologicaly 'sound', was empirically seriously flawed. So began the process of developing a dialogue between theoretical orientations and the representations of the lived experiences of my interviewees. That dialogue also involved developing fresh ideas about what constitutes being female in late 20th century Australian society. My own experience had been circumscribed by a critical academic discourse which privileged the rational and the 'outside' world, where the first person was never used and emotions, intuition and the 'inner' world were seen as inappropriate subject material for serious research.

I recruited my interviewees through my role as a telephone counsellor for an eating disorders self-help group. I asked every fifth caller, at the end of the counselling session, whether they would be interested in taking part in a piece of research to explore in detail the perceptions of people with eating disorders. I received a 100% response rate. All of those approached felt relieved that there was some way that they could reciprocate the time and energy that I had given them. We thus set up a democratic social contract where both parties gained from the relationship. In some cases the interviews were face to face, in others the interviewees preferred to remain anonymous and were interviewed over the telephone.

The contract with my interviewees involved providing a 'caring ear', listening to their problems and encouraging and supporting them in their attempts to resolve those problems. They in return provided me with insights into the problems that they experienced being female in a world that privileged the male. This contract situation proved most satisfying on both sides. My interviewees felt that they could not only reciprocate my efforts but that they could feel empowered by their perspective being taken seriously. I benefitted enormously by gaining insights into the way women who had been socialized outside of the critical academic tradition viewed the world. They, in fact, taught me what it is to be an embodiment of the feminine.

These insights into the unique experiences of women, however, did not give me a complete answer to the question: 'How is it that in some particular cultures, at a particular point in time, eating disorders appear in epidemic proportions?' In fact I needed to establish right from the start whether such an epidemic existed or whether it was an artefact of cultural and diagnostic processes. I thus developed an approach which was both theoretically and methodologically eclectic, using different theoretical and methodological traditions at the various levels of analysis.

The phenomenological theoretical tradition (Husserl, 1952; Binswanger, 1958; Merleau-Ponty, 1962) combined with the 'new' feminist theorists (Cixous, 1976; Irigaray 1985; Kristeva, 1986; Daly, 1987) provided a framework to develop methods for tapping the lived experience of people with anorexia and bulimia. The auto-biographical accounts of authors like Sheila MacLeod and the works of feminist writers in the area such as Marilyn Lawrence and Susie Orbach enriched the field from which the interview programme was devised. Helen Roberts' and Anne Oakley's writings were sources of constant inspiration at the interviewing stage of the research.

The political economy of health tradition (Doyal and Pennel, 1979; Navarro, 1983) inspired the development of a framework for examining the role of consumption in post-industrial Western societies and the economic role of the fashion, food, weight reduction, exercise and diet industries in helping to set the agenda for a rise in eating disorders. The macro-level of research was supplemented with cultural analysis and an examination of the role of patriarchal as well as economic social relations in circumscribing the choices available for women.

The work of Foucault and those who have used Foucault (Bordo, 1988; Celermajer, 1987; White and Epston, 1989) provided a backdrop for analysing the extent to which the micro- and macro-levels of analysis come together. The extent to which the anatomo-politics of individuals is reflected in the bio-politics of populations was examined through Bordo's (1988) work on anorexia as a 'crystallization' of societal disorder and Celermajer's (1987) analysis of anorexia as resistance to, rather than compliance with the social order.

In researching women's health it is important to use the sociological imagination in defining the 'problem' under investigation, in deciding on appropriate theoretical and methodological frameworks and in developing techniques to find answers to the problems posed (Mills, 1970). Slavish adherence to one particular methodological tradition stymies the imagination and may render the research politically sterile.

REFERENCES

Arndt, B. (1992) Proudfoot Saga has a twist or two, *The Weekend Australian* 15–16 Feb: Review 14.
Australian Institute of Health (1988) *Women's Health Data Requirements*, Australian Government Publishing Service (AGPS), Canberra.
Australian Institute of Health (1990) *Australia's Health 1990*, AGPS, Canberra.
Bates, E. and Linder-Pelz, S. (1990) *Health care issues*, revised edn, Allen & Unwin, Sydney.
Binswanger, L. (1958) The case of Ellen West, in *Existence* (eds R. May *et al.*) Basic Books, New York.
Bordo, S. (1988) Anorexia Nervosa: Psychopathology as the Crystallization of Culture, in *Feminism and Foucault: Reflections on Resistance* (eds I. Diamond and L. Quinby), Northeastern University Press, Boston.
Boston Women's Health Book Collective (1971) *Our Bodies, Ourselves*, Simon & Schuster, New York.
Broom, D.H. (1989) Masculine medicine, feminine illness: gender and health, in *Sociology of Health and Illness: Australian Readings* (eds G. Lupton and J. Najman) Macmillan, Melbourne.
Broom, D. (1990) *Research Priorities in Women's Health*, report to the Policy Development Division, Commonwealth Dept. Community Services and Health AYPS, Canberra.
Broom, D.H. (1991) *Damned if We Do: Contradictions in Women's Health Care*, Allen & Unwin, Sydney.
Brown, R.G.S. (1976) Social causes of disease, in *An Introduction to Medical Sociology* (ed. D. Tuckett), Tavistock, London.
Bryman, A. (1984) The debate about quantitative and qualitative research: a question of method or epistemology, *British Journal of Sociology*, **XXXV** (1), pp. 75–92.
Celermajer, D. (1987) Submission and rebellion: anorexia and a feminism of the body, *Australian Feminist Studies*, Summer (5), pp. 57–70.
Cixous, H. (1976) The laugh of Medusa, *Signs*, **1** (4), p. 835.
Commonwealth Dept. Health (1985) *Australian Women: A Health Perspective, A Summary of Statistical Indicators*, Australian Government Publishing Service, Canberra.
Commonwealth Dept. Community Services and Health (1989) *National Women's Health Policy: Advancing Women's Health in Australia*, AGPS, Canberra.
Davis, A. and George, J. (1988) *States of Health*, Harper & Row, New York.
Daly, M. (1982) *Gyn/Ecology*, The Women's Press, London.
Devault, M.L. (1990) Talking and listening from women's standpoint: feminist strategies for interviewing and analysis, *Social Problems*, **37** (1), pp. 96–116.
Dixon, J. (1990) Research debates and dilemmas: the feminist researcher as collaborator and strategist, paper to Women and Surgery Conference, Melbourne.

Doyal, L. and Pennel, I. (1979) *The Political Economy of Health*, Pluto, London.

Eckermann, E. (1987) Selfhood versus sainthood, in *Eating Disorders & Disordered Eating* (eds S. Abraham and D. Llewellyn-Jones), Ashwood House, Sydney.

Eckermann, E. (1991) Selfhood versus sainthood: towards a social conception of eating disorders, PhD thesis, Flinders University of South Australia.

Furler, E. (1985) Women and health: radical prevention, *New Doctor*, **37**, pp. 5–8.

Gardner, H. (ed.) (1992) *Health Policy: Development, Implementation and Evaluation in Australia*, Churchill Livingstone, Melbourne.

Healthsharing Women (1990) *The Healthsharing reader: Women Speak about Health*, Pandora, Sydney.

Hunt, L. (1991) The Women's Health Movement: A Study of a Solution, paper to the Australian Sociological Association Conference, Murdoch University, Perth.

Husserl, E. (1952) *Ideas* (trans. W.R.B. Gibson), Allen & Unwin, New York.

Kandal, T.R. (1988) *The Woman Question in Classical Sociological Theory*, International University Press, Miami, Florida.

Irigaray, L. (1985) *Speculum of the Other Woman*, Cornell University Press, New York.

Kane, P. (1991) *Researching Women's Health: An Issues Paper for the Department Health, Housing and Community Services*, AGPS, Canberra.

Kingston, M. (1991) Challenge in court to health plan 'sex bias'. *The Melbourne Age*, 1 March, p. 3.

Kristeva, J. (1986) *The Kristeva Reader* (ed. Coril Moi), Blackwell, Oxford.

Lofland, J. (1976) *Doing Social Life*, Wiley, New York.

Lupton, G. and Najman, J. (1989) *Sociology of Health and Illness*, Macmillan, New York.

McBride, A.B. and McBride, W.L. (1981) Theoretical underpinnings for women's health, *Women and Health*, **6** (1/2), pp. 37–55.

Meekosha, H. (1989) Research and the state: dilemmas of feminist practice, *Australian Journal of Social Issues*, **24** (4), pp. 249–68.

Merleau-Ponty, M. (1962) *Phenomenology of Perception*, Routledge & Kegan Paul, London.

Miller, M. (1986) Women and health: community development, its role in health: the future of public health research in Australia, *Community Health Studies*, **X** (4), pp. 417–8.

Mills, C. Wright (1970) *The Sociological Imagination*, Pelican Books, London.

Mitchell, J. and Oakley, A. (eds) (1986) *What is feminism?* Blackwell, Oxford.

Navarro, V. (1983) Radicalism, Marxism and medicine, *International Journal of Health Services*, **12**, pp. 179–202.

Oakley, A. (1981) Interviewing women: a contradiction in terms, in *Doing Feminist Research* (ed. H. Roberts), Routledge, London, pp. 30–61.

Orbach, S. (1985) Visibility/invisibility: social considerations in anorexia nervosa – a feminist perspective, in *Theory and Treatment of Anorexia Nervosa and Bulimia* (ed. S.W. Emmett), Brunner Mazel, New York.

Palmer, G. and Short, S. (1989) *Health Care and Public Policy: An Australian Analysis*, Macmillan, Melbourne.

Parsons, T. (1951) *The Social System*, Glencoe Free Press, London.

Parsons, T. (1964) *Social Structure and Personality*, Glencoe Free Press, London.

Roberts, H. (ed.) (1981) *Doing Feminist Research*, Routledge, London.

Saltman, D. (1991) *Women and Health: An Introduction to Issues*, Harcourt Brace Jovanovich, Sydney.

Schofield, T. (1990a) Collaborative research with community-based women's health organizations: a case study, paper to *Women and Surgery Conference*, Melbourne.

Schofield, T. (1990b) Feminism and women's health research: the experience of the Cumberland Centre for Women's Health Studies', paper to National Women's Conference, Canberra.

Short, L. (1992) Women are so stupid: that's why they need mammography, in *Women's Health in Australia* (ed. A. Smith), 2nd edn, University of New England, Armidale.

Smith, A. (ed.) (1992) *Women's Health in Australia*, 2nd edn., University of New England, Armidale.

South Australian Health Commission (1990) *A Social Health Atlas of South Australia*, South Australian Health Commission.

Stacey, J. and Thorne, B. (1985) The missing feminist revolution in sociology, *Social Problems*, **32** (4), pp. 310–16.

Turner, B.S. (1987) *Medical Power and Social Knowledge*, Sage, London.

Victorian Ministerial Women's Health Working Party (1987) *Why Women's Health?* Melbourne Health Department, Victoria.

Wadsworth, Y. (1984) *Do it Yourself Social Research*, Victoria Council Social Services.

Wass, A. (1992) The new legitimacy of women's health services – in whose interests? in *Women's health in Australia* (ed. A. Smith), 2nd edn, University of England, Armidale.

White, M. and Epston, D. (1989) *Literate Means to Therapeutic Ends*, Dulwich Centre Publishing, Adelaide.

Index